Rest Bites

First-Time Mums Guide to Finding Nurturing Rest & Rejuvenation

Written with Love
by Lucie Mala

Copyright © 2023 by Lucie Mala

All rights reserved.

No part of this book may be reproduced in any form or by any electronic or mechanical means, including information storage and retrieval systems, without written permission from the author, except for the use of brief quotations in a book review.

Disclaimer:

Although I am a massage therapist and a Yoga instructor, the content of this book is intended for information purposes only, it is not intended to diagnose, treat, cure, or prevent any conditions or disease. Please consult a physician before practicing the guided techniques in this book. Neither the publisher nor the author is engaged in rendering professional advice or services to the reader. The ideas and suggestions provided in this book are not intended as a substitute for seeking professional guidance. Neither the author nor the publisher shall be held responsible for any loss or damage allegedly arising from any suggestion or information contained in this book. The information presented is the author's opinion and does not constitute medical advice.

For all new mums.
Take care of yourself. That Love Bundle needs you.

Table of Contents

Foreword 9

Introduction 13
   How To Use This Book 19

Chapter 1 Once Upon A Sleepless Night 21
   The Sleep Dilemma 23

Chapter 2 Don't Mess With My Stress 61
   Parenting Stress 63

Chapter 3 Self-Care Is Not Optional, Mama 81
   What Is Self-Care? 85
   Self-Care Rituals You Can Start
   Implementing Today 88
   How To Make Self-Care A Part Of Your Life 93

Chapter 4 Mind To The Rescue 97
   The History And Science
   Behind Meditation And Mindfulness 99
   The Important Connection Between
   Breathing And Feeling In Control 103
   Clinically Proven Benefits: How Meditation
   Can Impact Various Aspects Of Your Life 105

Simple, Effective, Busy-Mum Proof
Meditation Exercises 112

Chapter 5 The Power Of Touch 125
Forgotten Wisdom: Massage Therapy
In Ancient Times..126
The Benefits Of Touch 129
How Engaging In Self- Massage Can
Save The Day..131
Self-Massage Rituals To Enrich
Your Life...134

Chapter 6 The Power Of Acupressure 147
What Is Acupressure? 147
The Origins And History
Of Acupuncture And Acupressure 149
All Mums Can Do With A Healthy
Amount Of Energy 151
How To Locate Your Body's Acupoints......................154
How To Practise Self-Acupressure................................156
Final Thoughts On Self-Acupressure......................... 189

Chapter 7 Restorative Yoga For Rest...................... 191
What Is Yoga? 191
A Brief History Of Yoga..192
Benefits Of Practising Yoga 192
The Best Type Of Yoga For Mums 193

Chapter 8 Yogic Sleep To The Rescue 235
From Grumpy To Chilled Mama In 30 Minutes 235

What Is Yoga Nidra? 236
The History Of Yoga Nidra 239
How Yoga Nidra Helps You
Sleep Better & Other Benefits 241
Guided Yoga Nidra Practise 243

Conclusion 249

About the Author 255

Bibliography 257

Foreword

The fact is that this book is more of a revelatory statement than a self-help book for mothers. To take rest seriously and study how to implement it in your life, in these times of overwhelm and over stimulation is an act of sheer revolution.

Yes, Lucie Mala is a quiet revolutionary, she has been spreading her message and kindness through the various communities which have been lucky enough to have her, and finally, finally, she has written down some of the tricks, treasures, and small miracles that can lead a mother, first time or otherwise into a more balanced state of being.

Medicine can be as complicated as you make it. Ultimately after over two decades of clinical practice, the obvious and mundane have become evident to me as the heart and soul of living well. If you don't rest you don't heal, recover, or recharge. Activity must be matched by rest or there is a cost, a bill that will have to be paid. As a physician, I have been helping people balance their books for a long time. I will forever welcome grounded, practical, and time-tested methods of moving the internal state into a restful place, and this is the reason for my wholehearted endorsement of *Rest Bites*.

The value of this book is that it gives in every sense and to every sense. You can read it and treat it as you feel fit for your life. Front to back, dip in, dip out, or as a gateway to deeper practice and exploration. This book heals, teaches, and guides mothers. There is no finger-wagging or judgement and no lofty ideals beyond the reach of typical family life.

This book is a companion. Lucie Mala has trodden the path of healer for a long time, and when she became a mother herself it was an obvious step and blessing for her to apply those skills and lay them down. *Rest Bites* is that blessing and gift for the community I know she values so deeply, modern mothers.

There is something fresh here, something that has truth and experience shining through it. The words and teachings in this book are hard-earned and speak with the warmth and compassion common to any great healer.

I know this book was informed and influenced by a big world, the world that shaped Lucie Mala. Decades ago you would have met her on small back roads in Africa, learning and travelling in the old ways, no internet or phones. She was driven on to learn and share, always has been and always will be. From Thailand way back in remote Buddhist Monasteries to her roots in Eastern Europe, Lucie sits quietly, brimming with the power and knowledge of a lifetime of following a passion. An unassuming sort, Lucie has always let her work do the talking. Never one to claim mastery or foster celebrity, Lucie has always respected traditional methods. She has studied many practices over the last two decades, and as with most true masters, the more she learns the more she has returned to the simple, and potent.

Lucie Mala has been through the initiation of childbirth just as you have, and now she has come full circle as a different being, with the same mission. In her face and in her words, you will see yourself reflected, whatever is with you will find a strong and loving companion. She has done her work and some of it, just some of it is here, captured in these pages. Hold it close.

Dr Andrew Smith, MBBS MRCGP
(GP, Medical consultant, and Acupuncturist)

***

Connect with Lucie on Instagram @the_rest_bites or on her website at TheRestBites.com.

Use the space below to write down any thoughts or feelings you are experiencing right now. Be sure to add a date so you can see how much you've grown as a person when you come across this page in the future.

Introduction

Ah, motherhood.

Those eyes. That teeny, boop-worthy nose. The smiles, the laughter, the irresistibly cute, silly moments. Aren't they just perfect?

If only you could enjoy your baby and every special moment with him or her to the fullest—without that little voice nagging inside. You know, the one yelling, 'I am SO tired!'

Do you faintly recall what it felt like to have energy? Do you hallucinate about a time this merciless onslaught of exhaustion didn't weigh you down? Are you kind of scared that you will never, ever experience those glory days again?

Oh, no...

Did you just feel a pang of guilt for daring to think there were better days before your little, joyous love bundle left the safety of your belly?

It's OK. You're not a terrible person. Everything you're feeling—good and bad—is normal. These are typical new-mum experiences. Few first-time mums talk about these things, because, well… it's damn hard to admit that we're not perfect.

Besides, between wanting to prove to your partner, the in-laws, and your parents that you've got this, putting on the best performance when visitors show up (who knew you knew so many people, right?), smiling through gritted teeth when people (yes, even those who don't have their own children) advise you on how to mother, and trying not to take mum-shaming personally.

But none of those issues compare to the unrelenting tiredness—it's a nightmare.

In fact, if it weren't for the tiredness, you would have enough mental and emotional perspective to distance yourself from issues like the ones mentioned above and not let them overwhelm you. You are a strong, resourceful woman, after all. You may not feel like it now, but you possess remarkable resilience and are capable of dealing with almost anything life throws at you.

But to harness the power of your resilience, you must invest in your own well-being just as much as you're investing in your child's well-being.

This book will empower you to take back control by teaching you how to find moments of deep, effective rest through simple techniques, all while being a full-time supermum. To give your absolute best to your newborn (or toddler), you need to take care of yourself first. You need to heed your body and mind's desire to feel nourished and cared for.

Take it from a mum who has been where you are now. If you neglect yourself, you will neglect those closest to you in one way or another.

- If you have a partner, you might appear distracted and disinterested in his thoughts, feelings, and experience of welcoming a child into your life. This may appear insensitive on your part and cause unnecessary friction in your relationship. Keep in mind that your partner loves you and wants to support you in the best way possible, but he cannot fully understand how the mental, emotional, and physical changes you went through (and are still going through) affect you. It's difficult to be sensitive to this fact when you're so tired. Extreme fatigue causes increased agitation that can make your reactions unpredictable at times. And before you know it, your partner becomes your unintended venting target. With the help of this book, you can regain your focus and patience, which will enable you to strengthen your bond with your partner and have the energy to take on daily challenges with vigour.

- Your family might feel you're pushing them away after they had supported you during your pregnancy. Once upon a time, you savoured every opportunity you had to spend time with your family. You adored them. These days, not so much. Their frequent calls, requests to visit, and well-meaning pep talks are nice and all, but it's annoying. This incomprehensible aversion to your loved ones has a lot to do with your stress-inducing fatigue. Although it's crucial that they give you the space you need to bond with your baby and adjust to a new way of life (or to raise your toddler the way you know is best), the family members you have healthy relationships with are also your allies and can assist in many ways. This book will help you understand how stress affects you, your children, and the rest of the family. You'll also learn to recognise stress symptoms and how to manage stress before it can overwhelm you.

- You might miss out on precious moments with your child because you are too exhausted to pay attention. As daunting as these days feel, you will look back not too long from now and wonder when and how your innocent, helpless baby became a walking, talking person. Every moment you have now with your child is fleeting and irreplaceable, so you owe it to yourself to be in the moment at all times.

Meet the Author Behind Rest Bites

I'm Lucie Mala, a fellow mum who has fallen, risen, learned, and conquered the tiresome woes of motherhood. Through this book, I want to help you navigate this exciting journey with more ease.

With a background in massage therapy, acupressure, yoga therapy, mindfulness meditation, and thousands of hours of working with new mums, I have a wealth of knowledge to share with you. The advice you'll find in these pages comes from my personal experience, as well as my experience of working with other mums who have all had their share of this weird, wonderful, and sometimes (OK—mostly) terrifying thing called motherhood.

As a busy, city-dwelling mother and therapist working with people on a daily basis, I have had to develop self-care routines to help me continually exude nurturing energy to provide the best service to my clients, all the while preventing myself from experiencing burnout at work and at home.

Having been through many highs and lows, I have grown passionate about empowering other women to reclaim their sanity and experience renewed energy. Kindness and love toward yourself are powerful catalysts for achieving a state of mind where you can feel calm and in control.

From my own experiences and testimonials from other mums, I have discovered our common enemy: exhaustion.

Almost all the stresses of motherhood can be traced back to this single factor. But, as every little prince and princess knows, enemies are there to be defeated. While I do not claim to have all the answers, I do know the difference that regular, meaningful rest breaks will make in your life. And that's why I want to empower you to live a more fulfilled life by introducing the techniques I teach other mums and also use myself. In fact, people have been using these techniques for thousands of years as a means of finding inner peace and understanding themselves on a deeper level.

I know exactly what you're going through. But more importantly, I know how to help.

I have lived through the same struggles of feeling lost because I didn't know how to rest or nourish myself when there was so little time in each day. However, in time, I developed effective mental tools and coping mechanisms to overcome the exhaustion. Once that happened, all the other aspects of motherhood became less intimidating and burdensome.

Friends and acquaintances soon noticed the changes in my life and begged me to share my secrets. After helping them, I realised I couldn't stop there, and that's why you're reading these words. The book you're holding is a result of my passion for women's health and well-being, as well as my intense desire to let other mums know there *is* hope.

I believe all mothers deserve to enjoy the blessing and beauty of motherhood with an abundance of energy.

How To Use This Book

The book is structured in such a way that you can dip in and out whenever you get a chance. There is no chronological order and no right or wrong way to approach the content. Wherever you open it, you will find a little rest bite, ready to feed your tired soul and give you whatever you need most at that moment. These rest bites may come in the form of words of encouragement, inspiration, support, and care, or an invitation to participate in a 5–15 minute exercise to rejuvenate yourself.

The words on these pages will not give you 'quick fixes' with no lasting effects. Instead, this is a guide to help you form new, lifelong habits that will become second nature to help you avoid distractions, live in the moment, and enjoy high energy levels every day.

Although you'll come across information backed by scientific research, you will find every sentence easy and fun to read.

Motherhood is wonderful and magical and filled with precious experiences. But it's hard and exhausting and frightening, too. So, don't be harsh on yourself if you feel like you don't know what you are doing right now. Rather, embrace the fact that this is all new territory in your life's journey, welcome the change, and see this time as an opportunity to grow as a person and first-time mother.

Above all, realise that you are not alone.

Whenever you open this book, you will feel empathetic, supportive hands reaching out to give you the advice you need. Here, no one will judge you or tell you what you should and shouldn't do. You'll find comfort and friendship from a fellow mum who has suffered just as much as you, who has found a way out of hopelessness, and who wants to show you that way.

Ultimately, this book is a testimony to you—the mother who conquered her fears and gave her children the very best of herself. Think of this book as a gift from the future you. It contains what you need: the secret to beating that unwelcome, overwhelming exhaustion that's stealing your joy.

It's time to take back your life, one little rest bite at a time. All you have to do is love yourself enough to take action.

Chapter 1
Once Upon A Sleepless Night

"Your life is about to change", said Gran.

"I know", I replied with a patient smile.

"It's going to be drastic. Nothing will be the same again…" Sister-in-Law added.

"I know…" I said with another smile, keeping a half-annoyed eye roll at bay.

"You're going to be tired; really, really tired—like nothing you've experienced before", Mum said in a caring tone as wisdom shone through her eyes.

I took both her hands in mine and asserted, "I know."

Mum glanced over at Gran, who winked at her. Then her gaze shifted to Sister-in-Law, whose smile seemed to say, "She has no clue…"

Despite the compassionate warnings of grandmothers, mothers, sisters, aunts, friends, and the occasional acquaintance, most women assume they'll be spared from the radical changes they'll inevitably face.

Granted, most of us experienced mental and physical changes during our pregnancies. I'm sure you can relate to one or more of the following changes I experienced:

bathrooms became my new best friends as the growing baby battled with my bladder for space;

sleep dwindled as the bump grew larger, and comfortable sleeping positions evaded me, despite the giant pillow between my legs;

mixed excitement and anxiety over the coming birth, meeting my precious baby, and pondering how I would adjust to a new way of life kept me wide awake as I envied my partner's deep, peaceful breathing next to me in the middle of the night;

and don't get me started on the leg cramps, heartburn, and... you probably have a plethora of things to add to the list.

With all *that* going on, how much worse could it get, right?

At this point, I have a confession to make. As a self-care practitioner who already specialised in the art of helping people feel relaxed, peaceful, supported, nourished, and restful before I got pregnant, I kind of had a chip on my shoulder. I figured, thanks to my occupation, I had the advantage of knowing how to stay in control in the midst of whatever life could throw at me. I was ready for that baby...

I was so ready that the moment the first bouts of extreme fatigue hit me after bringing my son home, I wanted to crawl into the foetal positions and cry, 'I'm not ready for this!'

The truth is, it doesn't matter how much you know, how many books you read, how many websites you consult, how many podcasts you listen to, how much advice you receive from your own mother or other, wiser women than yourself... nothing—as in nothing—can fully prepare you for the personal challenges of welcoming a precious new soul into your home. Your experience is, and will continue to be, unique. There is no single resource out there that will give you the answers to everything.

This is real life, and we learn as we go. However, there is one aspect of this rollercoaster ride called motherhood I can help you with, and that is fighting the exhaustion so that you can reclaim your energy and take on each day with a clear mind.

The Sleep Dilemma

Right now, your life feels upside down.

You should know, though, that nothing can flip life the 'right side up' for you, because there is nothing to flip. The crucial thing new parents miss is that when your baby becomes a part of the family, there is no turning back. Things will never, ever be the same again. Having a child enriches your existence in a way no parent can describe—why would you *want* to turn back?

While one night's proper rest may feel like a justifiable reason at this stage, it would be an impractical one. You'd return to your new life refreshed for a day, just to hear your brain nag, *'Warning... warning... low energy levels detected,'* long before the sun sets.

Wishful thinking is not the answer. But making sure you get your 8 hours of daily sleep with a baby in the house is not the answer, either; it's simply not possible for most new parents.

All you can do is adapt, and I'd like to give you the tools you need to do just that. I don't want to pressure you into accomplishing the impossible, especially if your baby has just joined the family. In the rest of this chapter, you and I will explore the science behind your and your baby's sleeping patterns. Then I'll show you how to make the most of your limited free time to rejuvenate yourself.

The Importance Of Sleep

People tend to think they can get away with little sleep. It's true that we're resilient and can adapt to less sleep than what we need when necessary, but this does not happen without consequences.

In this section, I want to help you understand why meaningful rest is important. People often neglect certain aspects of their lives because they're uninformed about the medium and long-term effects of said neglect. They justify not taking care of themselves because they feel fine —until they don't.

As a new mother, the exhaustion is overwhelming you. I know how you feel. I also know that despite the tiredness, grogginess, agitation, and depressing moments, sleeping is the last priority on your agenda (if it's a priority at all).

I'm not going to get preachy here and tell you to 'make sure you sleep at least 8 hours a night, otherwise…'

However, I want to share the science of how quality sleep affects your well-being. Hopefully, these facts will encourage you to implement the strategies I'll share during the course of this book. It is, after all, in your baby's best interest that your mental and physical health are at their best.

How Sleep Helps Your Mind And Body

When you sleep, your brain processes everything it has learned during the day. Its ability to adapt to what it learns is called brain plasticity, and it is this plasticity which has helped you develop your cognitive abilities and skills since childhood. However, without sleep, this ability diminishes, causing impaired learning and, thus, forgetfulness.

According to research, your brain uses the time you sleep to clear itself of toxins that have built up during the time you are awake. This is an interesting find, as the researchers of this study think there may be a direct link between poor sleep and increased cognitive impairment. The same study shows that your brain does not clean out toxins while you are awake, which is why sleep deprivation is dangerous. Brain cells are particularly sensitive and can suffer damage because of unchecked toxins. The same toxins can even interfere with your nerve functions and cause problems like delayed responses.

Further studies show that quality rest helps with your body's well-being, as your chances of developing high blood pressure and heart problems are less than when you suffer from long-term sleep deprivation. Your immune system also functions at its best when your body gets a chance to restore itself through sleep. This means you will be less likely to get infections and have the resources to fight off common illnesses like colds and influenza. A mind that enjoys proper rest is less likely to suffer from stress overload, too, which means you will be at less risk of developing depression.

The good news is that even with a new baby (or toddler) in the house, where regular, uninterrupted sleep is a pipe dream, all is not lost. Through my experiences and those of first-time mums I've worked with, I have discovered the secrets to giving your mind that much-needed rest without the luxury of long sleeping hours, all while enjoying the mental and physical benefits regular sleep provides.

To appreciate the power of the methods you'll learn, it's important to understand the cycles you go through when you sleep.

The Sleeping Cycle

Before the 1950s, the study of sleep was considered a boring topic by most scientists, because they believed our brains switch off while sleeping. But in 1951, Eugene Aserinksy would put that myth to rest and begin the fascinating field of studying brain activity while people sleep. Using his son to test (what was then considered) a clunky, old piece of equipment that supposedly tracked eye movements while he slept, Aserinksy stumbled upon the fact that our brains are very much awake while we sleep.

Today, thanks to the combined knowledge of those who specialise in the science behind sleep, we know that our brains use the sleepful state to recharge us for when we wake up and to maintain our bodies and repair damaged cells.

When you sleep, your brain takes you through cycles of 4 distinct stages throughout the night. When you have gone through all 4 stages, you have completed one sleeping cycle. A person will repeat the sleeping cycle several times a night. Each sleeping stage plays a role in how well you rest and whether you will wake up feeling refreshed in the morning.

The sleeping stages comprise two types of sleep:

- Non-Rapid Eye Movement (Non-REM or NREM) sleep.
- Rapid Eye Movement (REM) sleep.

Researchers have identified the different stages of sleep by studying neuron and brain wave activities in sleeping individuals. The first 3 of the 4 stages are spent in Non-REM sleep.

Stage 1

During the first stage, your brain uses a few minutes (typically no more than 5) to switch from a wakeful to a restful mode. Think of this as the lightest sleep you can enter. As you switch into restfulness, your heart rate and breathing slow, and your muscles relax but still twitch now and then. Your brain activity slows down slightly, but it is possible to wake easily from this stage of sleep. However, if left undisturbed, the transition into stage 2 happens fast.

Stage 2

In stage 2, a different pattern in your brain waves emerges. Your temperature drops, heart rate and breathing slow further, muscles relax to a point where they don't twitch anymore, and your eye movements stop. It also becomes harder to wake up from external stimuli such as background noise. During the first sleep cycle, stage 2 can last between 10 and 25 minutes and increase in length as the sleeping cycle repeats throughout the night. You spend up to half your night in this stage of sleep.

Stage 3

Also called delta sleep or short-wave sleep (SWS), stage 3 is the final stage of non-REM sleep before you enter REM sleep. It's called delta sleep because your brain waves make an identifiable pattern called delta waves. This is a state of deep sleep where your bodily functions like pulse, breathing, and muscle movements slow to their lowest levels. In this stage of sleep, it is hard to wake you.

Stage 3 sleep is the restful state you need most to wake up refreshed in the morning. The science of sleep is a fairly new field, but, as technology has progressed and scientists have gained a better understanding of how our brains work, we now know that the complete sleeping cycle is a dynamic biological system. Non-REM sleep and REM sleep serve different purposes, and you need both to function at your best. As people age, they spend less of their sleeping time in the deep-sleep phase.

During the first few rounds of sleep cycles, you experience stage 3 sleep at its best, with each stage lasting around 20 to 40 minutes. As the night progresses, you spend less time in this phase.

Stage 4

When you enter the 4th stage, known as REM sleep, your brain waves flare up to almost the same activity as when you are awake. This stage's most notable characteristic is the rapid movement of your eyes, which is where the term 'Rapid Eye Movement' comes from. Although you dream while in a deep sleep (stage 3), your dreams are most vivid during stage 4 of the sleep cycle. Other than your eyes' mobility and your breathing, your body is paralysed during REM-sleep to prevent you from acting out your dreams.

REM-sleep happens around 90 minutes after going to bed under normal circumstances. Your first REM-sleeping stage is the shortest, but it gets longer as the night progresses. You may spend as long as an hour in REM sleep in the later sleep cycles of the night.

Whereas deep sleep (stage 3 of non-REM sleep) is important for feeling fresh when you wake up, REM sleep enhances your learning ability, creativity, and memory.

Accept That Your Sleeping Cycle Is A Little Confused

Inadequate sleep, regular disruptions, and mild insomnia are now a part of your life.

Getting screamed awake in the middle of the night is not fun, but there is nothing better than knowing you are the source of everything and anything that little love bundle needs.

After your baby was born, your body continued on a hormonal rollercoaster ride. If you have recently given birth, enjoy the ride as best you can, because it's not over yet. After giving birth, your progesterone production reduces rapidly and takes its sleep-inducing properties with it. On top of that, as if someone is out to get you, your melatonin levels change. Melatonin is a hormone you produce as evening approaches and turns into a night to relax your mind and make you sleepy in preparation for bedtime.

Rest Bite Takeaway

Yes, the struggle is real, frustrating, and makes you emotional beyond description. But whatever you do, don't sigh in disappointment and give up on your own contentment—there is hope.

Talk with your partner and anyone else in your family you can trust. They can't support you if they're unsure of what you are experiencing. And remember that there are other first-time mums, probably not too far from you, who know exactly what you're going through. Don't underestimate the power of forming connections with like-minded people.

The sooner you accept that you will not enjoy a full night's rest for now, the better. As hard as it sounds, try to embrace the bad with the good of this phase in your child's life. Realise that even when life takes on a more regular routine, the exhaustion may not go away if you don't have effective techniques in place to fight it. Losing regular sleep is like losing the strength in your arm from disuse. If you want that strength back, you have to work the muscles in your arm. The ability to re-enter into re-energising sleep is no different. As you relearn how to use that valuable resource, you can rely on the powerful techniques you'll learn in this book.

Can't Get No Sleep Satisfaction

Every new mother's experience is different, but even with these differences, we're all tied by the same underlying challenges.

The 'baby blues' is a common occurrence among new mothers. It refers to shifts in your emotions that can last anywhere from a few hours up to 2 weeks after giving birth, and it affects up to 75% of new mums. Around 1 in 8 of those women will develop a more serious condition called postpartum depression.

If you experienced this, too, I'd like to emphasise that you have nothing to feel guilty over. There is nothing wrong with you. Sleep deprivation and postpartum depression are both natural consequences of welcoming a new life into the world.

Before my son arrived, everything seemed to be in order; I was under the impression that I had it all covered. The basics were sorted: there was enough income, and my husband, family, and friends had all pledged their support. Alas, none of that prevented my feelings of "baby blues" as the months after giving birth dragged on.

Like you, I realised my ability to focus, make good judgements, perform under pressure, and be creative took a serious beating. Of course, as mothers, we need these to be switched on and fully functioning at all times. Easier said than done, isn't it? It's impossible to describe how hard it is to juggle life and keep everyone happy as a new mum.

Podcasts encouraging rigorous self-affirmation regimes, love and support from loved ones, and strong cups of coffee helped a little. But these were ineffective distractions that could only divert my mind for minutes at a time.

Then, one fine day, frustrated and weepy, I let my guard down in an honest conversation with another mum I knew. It was both surprising and liberating to discover neither one of us was alone in our struggles. Whenever we observed each other before that day, we would think of each other as having everything under control. It was surprising and liberating to learn that we were fighting the same battle. It meant we now had the power to find a solution together. Through ongoing conversations, I learned that the number 1 problem both of us faced was that we were really, really tired. Being honest with myself gave me a deep desire to understand how extreme exhaustion was affecting my life and well-being.

Sleep Deprivation Can Worsen Postpartum Depression

Through my research, I learned that postpartum depression and sleep deprivation are tricky to distinguish and that the presence of one may intensify the other. In one study, researchers concluded that fatigue must be assessed whenever new mothers seek professional help. That said, there are various factors that doctors consider to diagnose postpartum depression.

While every mother's experience is different, be mindful of these tell-tale signs that you may have postpartum depression:

- losing interest in the things you normally enjoy;
- an inability to bond with your baby and feelings of guilt that you are a terrible mother;
- frequent crying, constant sadness, and mood swings.

If you are struggling with depression, the above symptoms will most likely be constant and last for days or weeks at a time. Note, however, that you may mistake sleep deprivation for depression. Since they share symptoms, it's best to steer clear of a self-diagnosis. Rather, consult a trusted practitioner if you suspect you may be suffering from more than extreme tiredness.

Your Partner Can Also Get Postpartum Depression

As mothers, we remain our babies' primary caregivers, especially if we breastfeed. This means it's natural that you will wake up more than your partner to tend to your baby's needs. Note, however, that although it might look like your partner is getting adequate rest, it's not necessarily the case.

More studies are being done to understand the effects of sleep deprivation in all aspects of people's lives. One team of researchers found a link between maternal and paternal depression. It seems that when mums are sleep deprived and develop depression, dads have a higher chance of developing depression, too.

> **Rest Bite Takeaway**
>
> While you may feel alone, know that your partner's life is also upside down. It's important that you keep an open, honest communication channel and do not feel scared or embarrassed to talk about what you are going through with your partner. If you open up, he will do the same.

No Bedroom Satisfaction

Don't blush; I know you know that I know. I won't discuss the details, but it is relevant to mention how sleep deprivation can affect intimacy with your partner. If your sex drive is out of order, rest assured, this, too, is a normal symptom of first-time mum sleeplessness.

Research on the relationship between sleep and sex is still new, but there is already evidence that they are linked. Think of them as partners: if one thrives, so does the other. The reverse is also true. Both are important to your health, as each can play a role in your emotional well-being, your relationship with your partner, and your quality of life in general.

The techniques I will share to help you feel more rested may increase your sexual drive. It could give you the opportunity to enjoy intimacy with your partner again and benefit your emotional well-being.

However, I am not a healthcare provider, and therefore I make no claims or guarantees that it will work for your sexuality. Please know that sexual dysfunction is a serious health concern, so be mindful of your own situation and reach out to a professional if your sex drive continues to evade you. Men and women of all ages are shy about talking about this issue and don't want to embarrass themselves. Just remember that many people struggle with their sexuality, so if this is an issue in your life, take solace in the knowledge that you're not alone. Do what you have to do to be there for your child and your partner, because taking care of yourself means taking care of them.

It Doesn't Have To Be This Way

There is a saying that knowledge is power. I couldn't agree more. After I learned and acknowledged that the root of my troubles was exhaustion, a strange feeling of empowerment settled over me.

I no longer felt helpless. Instead, I made the decision that I would not settle for a life where desperation for rest ruled the day. I wanted to be present in my life. I wanted to savour every moment with my son. I wanted to feel energetic and let all that energy radiate to my husband, baby, family and friends, and my clients. That's not to say the journey was easy, though.

Your journey won't feel like a stroll on a lazy afternoon, either. With the way you're feeling now, the results won't come quick enough. It's OK to get frustrated, but please don't give up. I know where you are, but I also know where you can be. Persist with me throughout this book, make the methods I share a part of your life, and you will experience the results you so desperately need.

Sleep deprivation can cause havoc in your life. If left unchecked, your body and mind will bombard you with more and more cries of distress in the form of physical pain, weight gain, more hormonal imbalances, and uncontrollable emotions. Eventually, you might lash out at the people who care about you most and experience trouble coping at work.

Your exhaustion is not your fault, but you do have the power to do something about it. In fact, just by reading these words, you've already shown that you are the kind of woman who will not sit yawning all day and live at the mercy of her sleeplessness.

Taking back control of your own sleep requires an understanding of how your baby's sleeping cycle works.

Your Baby's Sleeping Pattern

Few new parents consider the fact that a baby's sleep pattern differs from your own. When I learned about infant sleep patterns, it was as if some well-kept secret had been bestowed upon me. It gave me new hope.

An infant's sleep pattern is no secret, of course. It's just that the gravity of words like, 'Your baby is going to keep you up all night', don't sink in until we're immersed in reality.

On the other hand, I believe new parents don't receive enough scientific-based education about this phenomenon before their babies arrive. This is not your fault—neither pregnancies nor our love bundles come with instruction manuals. But it's never too late to learn about how babies sleep.

Talking about how well children sleep is a sensitive topic. The methods parents choose to approach this subject are varied. All things considered, I feel that I am in no position to advise you on this and trust that you are finding the right guidance and support if you are struggling with the process.

Instead of advising you on how to approach your child's sleeping habits, I want to highlight the typical sleeping pattern of babies, as this information was more valuable to me than receiving such advice on my own journey. In becoming aware of these patterns, I was able to appreciate my unique position more objectively. It helped me refrain from judging myself as an incompetent mother because I couldn't get my baby to sleep longer, and it gave me greater comfort during sleepless nights.

The body's ability to function in sync with the natural 24-hour daily cycle is called the circadian rhythm. Babies are not born with a fully functioning circadian rhythm. This is why they fall asleep and wake up at seemingly random times. In time, a baby develops a regular, more mature rhythm. How much sleep time he/she needs depends on various factors, of which the environment and his/her genes might play major roles.

Apart from their circadian rhythms being unsynchronised, babies' sleep cycles work a little differently from adult's. To better understand the difference between how you and your baby sleep, it helps to compare your sleep cycles. First, your own sleep cycles last 90–100 minutes, but your baby's cycle lasts around 50 minutes on average. While you cycle through the 4 stages of sleep in a predictable way under normal circumstances (1, 2, 3, 4, repeat), your baby experiences active or quiet sleep (the baby version of REM and non-REM sleep, respectively). In time, he/she will also go through 4 stages in his/her sleep cycles, but the length of his/her cycles will only match yours from around the age of five.

While you enter REM sleep during the last stage of your sleeping cycle and spend up to 20% of your sleeping time in that stage, your baby enters active sleep as soon as he/she falls asleep and spends 50–80% of his/her sleeping time in that phase. During REM sleep, your muscles cannot move, but in your baby's active sleep, he/she can stretch, wiggle, groan, and make the cutest faces and noises. This active sleep may be confusing. It's easy to think your baby is fussing and needs your help when, in fact, he/she's sound asleep. It helps to observe from a distance before you decide to pick up and soothe him/her, as he/she may not actually need it.

Babies spend most of their time sleeping, but because their internal clocks are still figuring out how the world works, they can wake up at any time to demand your loving attention. Most babies manage to sleep for at least 5 hours uninterrupted during the night by the age of 12 months, but it could happen sooner (or—as unappealing as it sounds —later).

If your love bundle is brand new, know that her sleeping pattern will become more stable when he/she is 3 or 4 months old. As he/she develops, this pattern may get interrupted, but it will be much easier for you to predict when he'll/she'll be awake or asleep than it is now. It may feel like the nightly interruptions will never end, but they will. In the coming months, your night rests will slowly get longer.

Your Baby's Inability To Sleep Through The Night Is A Blessing In Disguise

Active sleep in babies is a light sleep from which they can awaken easily, just like REM sleep in adults. Not many studies have been done to determine the role of REM (or active) sleep in babies. However, other studies have shown that REM sleep contributes to brain plasticity (the ability to continue learning) in adults. This has prompted studies into young brains, which seem to show that REM sleep contributes to babies' development through their visual experiences. According to Professor Marcos Frank, who initiated the studies, this may explain why babies spend so much more time in REM sleep than adults.

Sleeping light may protect babies from oxygen deprivation. If a person loses oxygen while asleep, she must be able to wake up as soon as possible. The same goes for babies. Light sleep ensures that their brains can respond fast to wake them up, whereas slower responses due to deep sleep may end in tragedy, like sudden infant death syndrome (SIDS). Discussing SIDS falls outside the scope of this book, but it is a risk you should be aware of, so please read up on it when you can.

Your baby's sleep pattern may not be ideal, but how she sleeps is crucial for her development and her safety. I hope learning about this from a scientific perspective has helped you gain a new appreciation in this regard. In any case, these restless days will end—maybe not soon enough, but sooner than you think.

Please, Please, Please Take Rest Seriously

You are a supermum, but even supermums need to recharge. You wouldn't be reading this if you did not agree. However, all mums are guilty of knowing they need to slow down, but still do nothing about it. We think anything and everything is more important—we'll sort ourselves out later.

Stop. Breathe.

If your baby could talk, he or she would say, 'Mama, you are my everything. I know I'm demanding, but that doesn't mean I don't want you to take care of yourself. My life depends on you, so please take some time to nurture yourself'.

Resting is a skill. If we don't practise it, we'll get rusty and suffer from sleep deprivation, which can lead to a host of terrible and terrifying mental and physical conditions. This is true whether children are involved or not, but it is a lot harder to master when a new life joins the family for the first time. Forming healthy, effective, and lasting resting habits is as much about mindset as it is about practise.

Let's Stop Wearing Busyness Like A Badge

When was the last time someone said to you, 'Oh, I'm doing great! I don't feel overwhelmed by everything I have to get done at all, so I feel relaxed—like I'm in control, you know?'

Modern life has tricked us into being busy bees. We feel left out or guilty if we don't say we're too busy, running around like crazy, or that we have SO much to do. It's as if taking a break has become something filthy that people look down on. Yet they live with constant dark rings under their eyes, they struggle to concentrate, preventable conditions like cardiovascular diseases prevail like it's a fashion trend, and despite their busyness, people never feel like they're getting things done.

Rest Bite Takeaway

Take a stand with me. Let's be societal rebels and defy expectations to set new standards for mums everywhere. Say no to endless busyness and give yourself permission to rest. This simple decision will have profound effects on your life. You'll feel less stressed, your creativity will blossom, you'll feel in control and balanced, and you'll feel more productive in the little time available to you.

Resting does not equate to 7 or 8 hours of daily sleep for new parents. It entails prioritising what's important to your well-being. Whether it's a simple indulgence like taking an essential-oil infused bath, or saying no when you're not up for social meetings, your body and mind will thank you for taking those short breaks.

To free yourself from the busyness mindset, incorporate the following into your life:

- be thankful for the little things that put a smile on your face;

- set 3 to 5 goals for every day and ignore all the other things you think you have to do;

- if you miss some daily goals, praise yourself for the ones you reached and don't scold yourself for the ones you didn't. You will learn to be more effective in task management as time passes;

- prioritise your goals to prevent feelings of overwhelm and unproductivity;

- choose simplicity and contentment; prioritise me-time and rest;

- include your partner in your decision to create balance and encourage him to do the same.

Intentional Rest—Your New Best Friend

You have at least 10–20 minutes to spare per day. You may be rolling your eyes or nodding your head to the little voice inside you saying, 'Whatever!' But it's true.

When I was first confronted with this idea, it seemed far-fetched. Whether you're a stay-at-home mum or a mum who needs to juggle family and office hours, there simply are not enough hours in the day. You need to clean the house, prepare food, do the laundry, check and answer emails, be in contact with the family, do that little favour for someone, and… just the thought of it all is exhausting, isn't it?

However, if you cultivate the new mindset we talked about in the above section, those precious 10–20 minutes will reveal themselves like magic. Most of the time, it will happen while your love bundle snoozes and recharges for his next round of play and mischief.

There is just 1 rule: when the 10–20-minute opportunity arises, prioritise yourself above all the 'should do's' and use it to form a habit of intentional rest. While it sounds easier said than done, it is possible and necessary. Any healthy habit takes time and perseverance to form, but once it becomes a part of you, it will be hard to imagine how you ever coped without it.

Research shows that taking a nap can give you a proper mental recharge without making you feel dazed when you wake up. I put this to the test and challenged the mums who come to me for therapy to do the same— it works wonders! Apart from increased energy, we experienced the following benefits:

- restored wakefulness, even as sleep-deprived mums (see Chapter 8);

- enhanced learning capability;

- increased performance in daily tasks; improved memory;

- lower blood pressure, which reduces the risk of developing heart and cognitive health issues; fewer mood swings.

If you can keep the timing of your naps consistent every day, you could eventually enjoy more time in the REM stage of sleep at night. This will have a restorative effect, thereby counteracting your sleep deprivation.

Keep Your Naps Short

Apart from significant benefits, the studies done on napping made an interesting find: napping too much is bad for you. Most adults get the most benefit from napping for 15–30 minutes. I have found that 20 minutes does the trick for most new mums.

That said, feel free to experiment so you can determine your optimal napping duration. It may be that you can get away with less than 20 minutes or that you need a little more time. Familiarise yourself with your baby's daily sleeping pattern, and then make sure you take your nap while he's/she's resting, too. His/her patterns will change, so be prepared to change your nap times as he/she develops. This is where setting those daily goals becomes helpful, because it will discourage you from engaging in 1 of the thousands of things you could do while your baby sleeps. Trust me, the wisest way to use your time while your baby or toddler doesn't require your attention is to restore your own energy levels. Remember that if you have a baby, he/she will nap many times throughout the day; you will use just one of those time slots to rest. For the remainder of the day, you can focus on your daily goals and do so with increased effectiveness. If your love bundle is a toddler, he/she will still take at least 1 nap, and that's your opportunity to take yours.

It's really important that your nap doesn't become a sleeping session. The moment you enter stage 3 of the sleeping cycle, you have gone too far and will wake up feeling groggy and even more tired for the rest of the day.

The Trouble With Excessive Napping

Napping for too long (lying down long enough to enter stages 3 and 4 of the sleep cycle) can aggravate your sleep deprivation and eventually result in a sleep disorder. Sleep disorders are detrimental and contribute to a host of mental and physical problems, including chronic pain and an increased risk of developing diabetes or heart problems.

Please be mindful of how you experience napping and how you behave before and after your naps. Once you make intentional rest a part of your daily routine and notice that you struggle to rise after naps, develop a desire to nap longer, or feel more exhausted than before your naps, reassess the time of day you nap, as well as how long you nap. You might even consider suspending your naps for a while.

It's also worth mentioning that if you find yourself growing more tired than usual during the day, you might have an undiagnosed medical condition or an existing one that is getting worse. However, napping may also become an unintentional escape from reality and the responsibilities of daily life. Life is incredibly stressful for new mums, so if this happens to you, the best decision would be to have a chat with your doctor about it. There is no shame in asking for help. Realising that you may have a problem and seeking help to change is brave and proves that you want the best for your family.

If taking naps is not possible for you, don't become discouraged. There are other restful techniques you can implement which will be just as effective. We'll talk about those in the upcoming chapters.

Sanity-Saving Bedtime Tips

One day, you'll cry from abundant laughter over the silly things you did when you first became a mother. You'll tell tales about the times you left the house half-dressed or constructed incomprehensible sentences like, 'If you don't get in the dishwasher now, we'll be late!'

For now, though, you'll have to go with the mummy-brain flow. Making intentional rest a part of your life will help you gain more control and have fewer of those moments. Intentional rest goes beyond taking naps to refresh your mind. An important part of making this habit effective entails a regime that gives you the best rest during your sleep-interrupted-filled nights. The following tips have spared many new mums' sanity.

Establish A Routine

It may seem like an impossible feat to establish a bedtime routine with a baby in the house. However, if you and your partner support each other in this endeavour, it will soon become a part of your life, and the benefits will make you happier and better-rested parents.

As your baby goes through his/her developmental stages, you may have to adjust your routine slightly, so it is important to remain flexible in this regard. He/she will, however, develop a routine with more ease from around the age of 6 months old. Some babies will not sleep for hours on end during the night until they're at least 12 months old. Work your bedtime routine around his/her sleep pattern until he/she is ready to sleep through. If your love bundle is older than a year, you can help him/her join in the new routine by getting him/her calm as bedtime approaches. Since every parenting style is unique, I will not advise you on how you can get your baby ready to sleep.

Step 1: Wind Down 40 Minutes To An Hour Before You Go To Sleep

As bedtime approaches, dim all the lights. If you can't dim them, switch off the main lights and keep only lamps switched on or burn a few candles.

Step 2: Switch Off The Digital Stuff

Check your mobile phone for the last time and leave it in a different room than the bedroom for the night, and switch off your computer or laptop. As a rule, avoid digital screens for at least half an hour before you want to sleep to get away from the blue light they emit.

Blue light has the highest energy level and shortest wavelength of all visible light the human eye can see. The sun is the primary source of blue light, which keeps you alert and helps boost your cognitive functions. In fact, natural blue light from the sun is crucial for your baby's developing eyes, as well as the health of your own eyes. Blue light also regulates your circadian rhythm. When the sun sets and the blue light disappears, your body prepares to switch off for the night by producing the sleep-inducing hormone melatonin.

However, modern digital screens also give off blue light, thus messing with your circadian rhythm. Your eyes cannot distinguish between natural blue light and artificial blue light produced by digital devices. When you continue to use your digital devices in the evening, your body cannot produce melatonin to make you sleepy. So, by the time you climb into bed, you are wide awake and will struggle to fall asleep. Of course, because life has a wicked sense of humour sometimes, your baby will probably cry by the time you finally doze off.

Step 3: Make Your Bedroom A Technology-Free Zone

Apart from blue light, digital devices also emit sounds that can disturb your sleep. It doesn't matter if you switch your mobile phone to silent, either, because if you wake up in the middle of the night, you'll probably want to check the time or browse on your favourite social media platform instead of trying to go back to sleep. If you really can't sleep again, read a book instead, as it will ease your mind and probably induce drowsiness.

Step 4: Practise At Least 1 Self-Care Ritual

In Chapters 4 to 8, I'll introduce you to effective self-care rituals that will help you relax, focus, and take care of yourself so you can beat your exhaustion and start to feel like yourself again. From self-acupressure to mindfulness techniques, you'll have an array of go-to techniques to help you regain your vigour.

Step 5: Check The Clock

Go to sleep at the same time every night, preferably between 21:30 and 22:30 (9:30 PM and 10:30 PM). This time range gives enough time for you to enjoy at least 1 full sleep cycle. As with your daytime naps, test which times work best. You'll know if the time you went to bed worked by how well rested and alert you feel when you wake up in the morning.

A bedtime routine is important, even if you have to wake up in the middle of the night. Helping your body find a rhythm so it knows when to produce melatonin (to make you sleepy at night) and when to produce cortisol (to make you alert during the day) will make you feel more relaxed and rested than without a routine. If you can get through at least one uninterrupted sleep cycle every night, you'll experience a significant change in your mood and ability to function during the day.

Take Epsom Salt Baths At Least Twice A Week

Epsom salt won't make your food taste great, but it is a miracle compound that has been used to treat various ailments since its discovery in the 17th century. It's called salt, not because of its compound or taste, but because of its chemical structure. Its name comes from Epsom, the English town where it was first discovered.

All you have to know, though, is that Epsom salt is a rich source of magnesium, a mineral essential for over 300 biochemical processes in your body. Your body needs magnesium to manage stress and to sleep properly. You can boost your body's magnesium levels by consuming magnesium-rich foods (such as collard greens, legumes, seeds, and nuts) and taking supplements.

However, I have found a brilliant excuse to laze in a steaming bath, all while enjoying the sleep-inducing benefits magnesium offers: an Epsom salt bath.

No conclusive studies have shown that the human body absorbs minerals like magnesium through the skin, but that has not stopped people, including healthcare professionals, from declaring the wonders of taking an Epsom salt bath.

New mums are willing to try almost anything to feel less exhausted, and I was no exception. While taking these baths did not turn me into Sleeping Beauty, I felt indescribably relaxed once I started incorporating it into my life. Of course, feeling more relaxed helped me fall asleep faster than before.

I'll admit that, more likely than not, the relaxation from taking Epsom salt baths has more to do with lovely, steaming water and enjoying personal time than an actual biochemical reaction that takes place. Either way, it works—so go ahead and try it.

You can even add essential oils to your bath, which are also known for their calming effects and ability to boost your immune system. A study proved that lavender essential oil can enhance non-REM slow and deep-wave sleep, which is just what you need to wake up feeling refreshed in the morning.

Take your baths in the winding down time frame just before bedtime for the best results.

Create A Restful Environment

If you can make your bedroom a technology-free zone like we discussed earlier, you're halfway there to experiencing better sleep. Here are more things I have done that helped me sleep better.

Keep Your Bedroom Clutter Free

There is a reason why 'declutter' is such a buzzword. It's not just the latest decor trend. Cleaning up your space flexes your decision-making skills, boosts your confidence, reduces anxiety, and makes for an enjoyable sleeping environment.

The Darker, The Better

Light tells your body that it should be alert and impedes your brain's melatonin production. If your bedroom gets too much light from the outside, consider installing blackout curtains. Also, if you use an alarm clock, either set its display brightness to the lowest setting or turn it away from facing you. If your mobile phone is your alarm clock, silence all notifications and put it as far away from the bed as possible, like on the dresser. With a decluttered room, there will be no risk of tripping over or bumping into things if you need to stand up to attend to your baby during the night.

Aromatherapy

Natural scents from essential oils can relax your mind and promote sleep. You already know that lavender is an excellent choice, but there are many scents to experiment with. Find the one that works for you and use it to enjoy quality rest at night.

Keep The Bedroom Cool

Temperature plays a major role in whether you sleep well or not. Heat exposure can decrease slow-wave sleep and promote wakefulness, so if you can, make sure your bedroom is cool at night. Comfortable temperatures range between 60–71 degrees Fahrenheit (15.6–22.0 degrees Celsius).

You Can Only Sleep As Well As The Quality Of Your Mattress

Few people consider the quality of their beds as a factor in how well they sleep, but in many cases, it is the number 1 reason people wake up exhausted. Your number 1 reason is your love bundle, but your mattress and pillow might just as well be the second major culprit.

A quality mattress and pillow support your skeletal structure and makes sure you do not wake up with body aches, which is the last thing new parents need. Investing in a proper bed should be a priority if you don't have one.

Give Your Body Proper Nutrients

The quality of your food determines the quality of your life. Numerous studies throughout the decades have proven that nutrition is the foundation of a healthy mind and body. While most people know that diet can affect their weight, blood sugar levels, and cholesterol, not many consider how their food intake influences how well they sleep.

There is no one diet to follow for better sleep. However, these general tips can make a remarkable difference in the quality of your sleep:

- eat foods rich in vitamins and minerals, like a large variety of vegetables and fruits;

- avoid consuming a lot of sugar (stay far, far away from those energy drinks); avoid junk food;

- don't eat meals close to bedtime;

- resist the temptation to snack late at night (but if you must, drink a cup of warm milk with a bit of honey for sweetness, as milk contains a sleep-inducing amino acid).

Sleep deprivation is a daunting reality for new mums and dads, but it is possible to counter its relentless effects with the right mindset and techniques. In this chapter, you learned about the science behind your own and your baby's sleep cycles, and you picked up handy tips to help you prioritise rest above everything else. As important as it is, proper sleep is just one part of the puzzle to combat fatigue. Next, we'll explore the role of stress to determine how it contributes to your exhaustion and how you can beat the blues.

> It's very important that we re-learn the art of resting and relaxing. Not only does it help prevent the onset of many illnesses that develop through chronic tension and worrying; it allows us to clear our minds, focus, and find creative solutions to problems.
>
> (Thich Nhat Hanh)

Use the space below to write down any thoughts or feelings you are experiencing right now. Be sure to add a date so you can see how much you've grown as a person when you come across this page in the future.

_____
_____
_____
_____
_____
_____
_____
_____
_____
_____
_____
_____
_____
_____
_____
_____
_____
_____

Chapter 2
Don't Mess With My Stress

Every mum has experienced an array of life's stresses that causes burnout. Of course, these situations happen in the midst of managing our careers, marriages and households, and raising our beautiful, curious, energetic children.

I know the guilt of losing patience at discovering yet another scribble on the wall. I know the comfort a glass of wine offers at the end of a torturous day—and the consequences it brings the following day. I know the intense pain of feeling alone, despite having people around you. I know how badly you want to lock yourself in a room and scream your lungs out on some days.

> ### Rest Bite Takeaway
>
> Whatever you are facing, realise that your frustrations are a part of the journey. As long as you accept each challenge as a lesson to help you become stronger, you'll always find a way to overcome it.

Through my trials, I have learned what serves me and my family best, and I want to pass that knowledge on to you. In the rest of this chapter, I'll share helpful methods to help you navigate the storm of motherhood with less stress to weigh you down and more inner peace to enjoy precious moments with your family.

**Stress May Be Ugly,
But It Reveals The Beauty Of Life**

The truth of life is that good and bad go hand-in-hand. You cannot have one without the other. Our human experience is a mixture of joy and despair, confidence and fear, happiness and sadness, and fun and boredom.

Here is an important lesson I've learned: the sky is at its prettiest just after a storm. This means that if it weren't for the ugly and bad experiences in life, no one would recognise the beautiful and wonderful experiences. Think back on your pregnancy. As that love bundle grew and fought for space, daily life became pretty uncomfortable. Carrying a growing baby is no easy feat, but if someone were to ask whether you would go through the stress again, I bet you'd answer with a resounding 'yes'. The reason is obvious—the amount of physical and mental exhaustion and pain of your pregnancy was totally worth meeting your child and experiencing the indescribable delight he or she has brought into your life.

Parenting Stress

The many challenges brought on by motherhood are natural. You can't avoid stress completely (trust me, mothers the world over have tried...), but you can choose a lifestyle that does not allow it to affect you and your family in a destructive way.

Of all the pressures you deal with, unchecked parenting stress is probably the most dangerous, because it has the power to influence and alter your love bundle's development.

I don't use 'dangerous' lightly, nor is it my intention to scare you. Instead, I want to talk about the effects of this kind of stress to empower you. In time, I discovered that there is a profound connection between parents and their children, called brain-to-brain synchrony, or parent-child synchrony. In this section, I'll walk you through what you can expect from parenting stress and how it affects caregiving.

What is Parenting Stress?

As the term suggests, parenting stress revolves around how well we cope as parents. When you feel you can't meet the unique challenges brought on by parenthood, parenting stress kicks in.

From internal to external factors, there are many things that can trigger parenting stress. Basically, if you perceive anything as threatening your ability to keep your child happy, safe, and healthy, you will very likely experience parenting stress. Of course, parents are always concerned about those things, so, in a sense, parenting stress is a given (even more so for a new mum).

As bleak as that sounds, you're in a much better position than a parent who is not even aware of this type of stress. When you're aware of a phenomenon and its consequences, it empowers you to work around it. Also, always keep in mind that feeling overwhelmed from mothering is no reflection on your parenting skills or your worthiness as a parent. In all honesty, if these things *didn't* worry you, you'd have something to feel guilty about! Don't allow negative thoughts like that to maul in your head, because it will only aggravate your stress levels.

Let's explore why parenting stress can have such profound implications for your love bundle.

Brain-To-Brain Synchrony Between You And Your Child

Brain-to-brain synchrony is nothing new. Studies have proven that when we're engaged in meaningful interactions with others, our brain waves match up with those of our peers.

When it comes to the neural-level connections between mums and babies, studies show that babies' brainwaves match those of their mothers when they make eye contact and their mothers talk to them.

Apart from that, if you are less stressed out and are engaged in an activity with your baby, your brain waves also move in sync. Conversely, if you experience high levels of stress, you tend to become less engaged in the activities you do with your baby, and this causes a difference in your and your baby's brain waves.

While more studies are required to fully understand the significance of brain-to-brain synchrony between mums and their babies, it's becoming more apparent that this is the means through which babies first learn to communicate and connect with other people.

The bond between mother and child is indeed powerful, and it's not just in our minds. Ruth Feldman, together with her colleagues, did experiments in which they discovered that mothers and their babies' heart rhythms matched up during face-to-face interactions that included happy sounds and non-verbal positive queues. Another experiment showed that babies are very much in tune with their mothers and can pick up when they're really stressed. In this experiment, mothers were asked to take part in a difficult task, after which they were reunited with their babies. Soon after being reunited, the babies mirrored their worried mothers' cardiac responses.

How Your Stress Can Affect You And Your Child

Research has been done on the consequences of being stressed out when you have kids. However, most mums (and dads) don't need studies to confirm what they've already experienced themselves. I've done it, and there is probably not a parent out there who has not done it:

- ◆ We overreact.

- ◆ We withdraw and shut down our emotions.

Does this make us incompetent parents? No, it simply makes us human. And being human, we have the capacity to learn from our mistakes and adapt our behaviours.

As mentioned in the *Brain-to-Brain Synchrony Between You and Your Child* section, there is strong evidence to suggest that our babies learn social behaviours through us. If your baby can't form a meaningful connection with you because you are stressed and distracted, he's going to have a hard time doing it with other people as he grows into his own person.

Your stress is not your fault, so you have nothing to be ashamed of here. All you need is loving guidance to make it stop. That is why I've poured all my knowledge of self-care for mums into this book. I want to give you all the tools you need to cope.

> The greatest weapon against stress is our ability to choose one thought over another.
>
> (William James)

Tips For Dealing With Parenting Stress.

Ask For Help

No, I'm not kidding. In my experience, new mums are notoriously bad at reaching out for a helping hand. It's normal to think doing so is a reflection of your capabilities as a mother, but it's not. It's the smart thing to do. Your grandmother has been there, your mother has been there, and now you're here. People need people in all aspects of life to thrive, and motherhood is no different. Think of it this way: would you want your son or daughter to reach out to you one day if they're having a difficult time?

Western culture has separated us from what our ancestors offered: support. Really, trying to go at it alone is a modern and unnecessary issue. If you don't have family and friends nearby to support you, reach out to parenting communities or befriend other mums in your area.

Whatever you do, do not try to do this alone. It's OK to need and ask for help.

Take A Stand Against Negative Influences

Whether it's a friend who complains about most things, negative news in the media, or bad memories, negative influences can make your stress worse. When you get exposed to positivity, your brain seeks out other positive experiences. It works the same when you get exposed to negativity.

If you feed your mind with negativity, thereby increasing your stress levels, you are at greater risk of making rash decisions, lashing out at the wrong people at the wrong time, and undermining your ability to solve problems rationally.

Do your best to avoid or at least limit negative influences in your life.

Avoid Time Pressure By Sticking To A Daily Schedule

In Chapter 1, I mentioned that you should have no more than 5 goals per day. To take the pressure off even more, you can schedule each day the evening before. Having structured days makes you feel more in control and motivates you to stick to that schedule. And, yes, it's totally possible to have a schedule with a baby in the house. I'm not saying things will always work out to a tee, but you'll be surprised at the difference this simple technique can make.

Practise Cognitive Empathy

To appreciate cognitive empathy, we have to contrast it with affective empathy.

Simply put, affective empathy is when you feel another's pain when they're unhappy. While being sensitive to others (especially your love bundle) is important, affective empathy can also cause you to overreact, thereby heightening your stress. Once that happens, the chances that you'll snap and use harsh words increase significantly.

Cognitive empathy, on the other hand, allows you to assess a situation objectively and come up with helpful solutions, all while showing you care. When you use cognitive empathy, you take an analytical approach by trying to see the situation from the other person's perspective and also thinking about the one thing that would make her feel better.

Practising cognitive empathy instead of affective empathy prevents you from living your child's pain and gives you the mental space to help her overcome that pain. Being objective about the issue does not make you insensitive. If anything, it empowers you to help your baby in the quickest way possible.

Find Inspiration

It is crucial to your well-being to still seek out experiences that result in personal fulfilment and add meaning to your life.

> **Rest Bite Takeaway**
>
> Your individuality did not cease to exist the moment your baby came home with you, so don't neglect what makes you happy and inspires you to live with abundance. If you continue to pursue things that make life more meaningful to you, you have a powerful weapon to fight against toxic stress. In turn, this will protect your mental health and give you the emotional space to strengthen bonds with your partner and your baby.

The Bright Side Of Stress

You may have heard this before, but not all stress is bad. When your baby cries, you become stressed. It is that stress that drives you to ease your baby's discomfort. When you're out in public, stress heightens your senses and allows you to react appropriately to threatening situations, like quickly stepping on your car's brake pedal when the vehicle in front of you halts. Then there is the stress that causes excitement without the feeling of being threatened, called 'eustress' like when you and your partner have a date night, when your baby achieves a milestone, or when you have a challenging project to complete.

A life without stress is like you without your child—it doesn't work. It plays an important role in helping you make the right decisions when needed and even adds flavour to what would otherwise be a rather boring existence. But a life with too much stress is, well... stressful.

The Not-So Bright Side Of Stress

While humans have the mental and physical resources to cope with healthy doses of stress, we suffer when it exceeds those resources. When we fail to recognise the signs our bodies give that the pressures of life are too much, overwhelm will take over and cause havoc in the form of physical and mental illness. People's busyness has led them to ignore their internal warning signs. At the same time, they're so caught up in their own lives that they don't realise when those close to them behave or look different than usual because of the things *they* have to deal with, too. This is true even in the same household, like a couple who has just welcomed a new life into the home. More often than not, people reach breaking point before anyone notices something is seriously wrong.

As a new mother, you are at greater risk of not noticing when your body tries to tell you that you are in danger of being overwhelmed by too much stress. Your exhaustion is, once again, a primary culprit. So, before we discuss how to deal with stress, let's talk about its effects and how to recognise when it's trying to take over your life.

Warning Signs That You're Under Too Much Pressure

First, I'd like to point out that no two people are the same. Stress is a personal experience, and each of us reacts differently to the same situations. For that reason, I won't go into what can cause unhealthy stress. Be honest with yourself as I discuss the following symptoms and then make a decision not to allow stress to rule your life because you are strong enough to overcome your difficulties. You simply need effective tools to deal with those difficulties so they will not hamper your happiness. As with busyness, people treat stress as if it's something to be proud of. If you have stepped into that trap, it's time to cut the noose and say, 'No more!'

Physical Tell-Tales Of Too Much Stress

Upset Stomach

Did you know that your digestive system contains 500 million neurons? The rest are in your brain and nervous system. In a sense, your gut is an extension of your brain, giving the infamous 'gut feeling' a whole new meaning. Your gut cells can produce serotonin (happy hormones) independently of your brain, and some microbes in your gut produce a neurotransmitter that contributes to the management of your feelings of fear and anxiety.

This makes it quite obvious why one of the most common symptoms of stress overwhelm is an upset stomach. You can experience diarrhoea, constipation, nausea, cramps, a loss of appetite or uncontrolled hunger, and heartburn.

Headaches and Other Body Aches

When stress gets on your nerves, it is likely to trigger a tension headache, characterised by pain around your neck, facial area, and head. These types of headaches are more annoying than dangerous. However, the problem is that when you can't deal with stress effectively, it creates a vicious cycle whereby stress leads to headaches, and headaches lead to more stress.

Constant body pain for no apparent reason is also a sign of chronic stress. Your body is designed to tense up muscles and prepare you to flee from dangerous situations. When the danger disappears, your body relaxes, and the pain from tensed-up muscles disappears. It's important to understand that your body reacts to threats, whether it is real (like when you have to dodge a moving object to avoid injury) or perceived (feeling overwhelmed from mothering, maintaining relationships, coping at work, etc.). From back pain to tender joints, your body will punish you when you don't keep your stress levels in check.

Compromised Immunity

Unchecked stress has a nasty friend—a hormone called cortisol. This hormone and your immune system don't get along. It has a particularly abusive relationship with lymphocytes, one of the many types of white blood cells. The stress hormone lowers the lymphocyte count in your body and hampers communication between white blood cells throughout your body, which makes it easy for bacterial and viral infections to slip in and make you ill.

Low Energy Levels And Insomnia

As if new mums aren't tired enough, stress can worsen the exhaustion. In this case, too, you can deal with a vicious cycle when you don't have effective ways to fight off stress. As with headaches, low energy levels and sleeplessness brought on by stress can cause you to become more stressed. This can lead to insomnia, a sleep disorder characterised by extreme difficulty falling asleep, maintaining sleep, and enjoying quality sleep.

Other Physical Symptoms Related To Stress

- Fast heart rate and chest pain.

- Constant fidgeting.

- Sweaty hands and feet.

- Shaking and nervousness.

- Trouble swallowing.

- A dry mouth.

- Grinding your teeth and clenching your jaw.

If you ask what is the single most important key to longevity, I would have to say it is avoiding worry, stress and tension. And if you didn't ask me, I'd still have to say it.

(George Burns)

Mental (Or Cognitive) Tell-Tales Of Too Much Stress

Poor Judgement

Research shows that people resort to binary, reactionary decision making under stress. As mums, we live under immense pressure because of all our responsibilities. When we don't counter those pressures with effective relaxation methods, it's all too easy to make poor decisions. When your decisions are reactionary, you fail to assess situations from an objective point of view and struggle to choose the best solutions. This often leaves you feeling inadequate and affects your self-esteem, which is an emotional symptom of stress, (we'll talk about self-esteem in a bit.)

Worrying, Negative, And Racing Thoughts

If stress hormones have been flooding your body for a while, you may notice that you feel anxious a lot and that your mind is full of 'what if' scenarios. It can escalate to a point where you have little to no control over racing thoughts that steal your attention when trying to accomplish important tasks. In time, constant worrying can influence your outlook on life into a pessimistic one. Chronic stress and anxiety are dangerous, as they can lead to an anxiety disorder, depression, and even dementia.

I cannot stress enough (pun intended) how important it is for you to listen to your mind and body and to start relaxing today. The solution to relieving the effects of stress is easier than you think, but I also want to encourage you to seek professional help if you feel like your situation has become unbearable.

Other Cognitive Symptoms Related to Stress

- Trouble focusing.

- Trouble remembering.

- A scattered, disorganised mind.

Emotional Tell-Tales Of Too Much Stress

Feeling Like You Have Lost Control

Every woman's life becomes more hectic when her love bundle joins the family. Add the cognitive effects of stress, and it soon results in getting fewer things done than what you're used to. It's disheartening to realise that your productivity isn't what it used to be, and it may leave the impression that you've lost control. In reality, though, the dynamics of your life have shifted, and you haven't adapted yet. The techniques I'll introduce in the following chapters will ease your transition into a new lifestyle with a child and help you accept that life has changed forever— for the better.

Low Self-Esteem

Worrying thoughts, believing that you've made a ton of wrong decisions, and feeling like life is spinning out of control are not healthy for anyone's confidence. As new mums, we're especially sensitive in this regard because we feel like we have so much to prove and don't want our partners and family members to think we're incompetent. Ironically, we're our own worst enemies in this case. We're so worried about how others perceive our mothering abilities that it leads to a false sense of incompetence when we look at ourselves in the mirror.

If you're a little hostile when you receive criticism and find yourself avoiding conversations with those closest to you, you may be suffering from low self-esteem.

Moodiness And Frustration

Not to be confused with signs of low self-esteem, moodiness refers to unpredictable reactions to seemingly normal events. When you suffer from too much stress, you can go from fairly calm to intensely agitated or sad enough to burst into tears in minutes. If little things are frustrating you all of a sudden, it's your mind telling you that it needs a well-deserved break.

Other Emotional Symptoms Related To Stress

- Depression.
- Trouble quieting inner criticism.
- Feeling indifferent or underwhelmed when you engage in activities that made you happy or excited in the past.

Be Grateful For Your Symptoms

Your body is an amazing biological machine, and it wants you to enjoy an abundant, stress-free, pain-free life. When symptoms like the ones we discussed above come knocking, treat them as warning signs that you need more balance. You're a new mum—this is supposed to be the happiest time of your life.

> ### Rest Bite Takeaway
>
> If you could show yourself just a fraction of the love your child has for you, you would realise how much you're worth and how much you deserve to take better care of yourself.

Once, I felt caged in by a limiting, unpleasant, and seemingly endless cycle of stress. It felt impossible to break free because I did not know how to help myself. But when I learned how to recognise stress symptoms and understood how stress affects me, I felt motivated, determined, and even excited to find creative, lasting ways to change the way I react to stress to get rid of its unwelcome effects.

If you feel stuck, I want you to know that it's OK. You'll be OK. If you've been harsh on yourself, it's time to make peace and let go. You've been doing your best, and you'll continue to do your best because you're a wonderful mother who wants the absolute best for her baby.

In the coming chapters, you will find a collection of strategies that have worked for all the mums who have visited my practice over the years. It is time to restore balance in your life. There is no particular order in the techniques I'll share, and some may appeal more to you than others. Take your time to read through each chapter, take notes on which self-care rituals you would like to start with, and then implement them as soon as yesterday. Don't make plans to do it—get started right away, because there is no better time to take back control than now.

It's not the load that breaks you down, it's the way you carry it.

(Lou Holtz)

Chapter 3
Self-Care Is Not Optional, Mama

Modern life is a tricky rascal. For all the conveniences it offers, it comes with just as many headaches. People are so busy being busy, so caught up stressing over this and that, and so distracted that they hardly notice when their bodies say, 'I need a break'.

Those who do notice shrug it off as symptoms of the times. Body aches, headaches, racing hearts, shaking hands, not remembering what you did a few minutes ago… These things are just a part of life, right?

Wrong!

You can only enjoy life, despite its many challenges, when you stop, listen, and react when your body communicates with you.

When your child cries, you want to do everything in your power to make his or her little life better. Treat your body and mind with the same care, and you'll be astonished at what you've been missing—even before you got pregnant.

Before I got into offering massage therapy and Yoga, I lived my life on autopilot mode. Without the knowledge I have today, I was detached from myself, unable to recognise the crucial connection between my body and mind. I intellectualised everything, lived in my head, and never noticed my own breathing. The idea that stress could manifest in the form of tight muscles, causing pain in places I'd never have imagined, was foreign to me. Above all, I felt helpless and, like so many women, stepped into the trap of accepting that whatever bodily ailments came my way was a part of being human. Deep inside, though, I was restless. Something about accepting that there was nothing I could do to feel stronger and more energised felt wrong. As time passed, I realised—decided, really—there had to be a less painful and stressful way to live.

Rest Bite Takeaway

The next time you see yourself in the mirror, pause and stare. Look deep into those eyes and remind yourself of how far you've come. You could never have accomplished anything in life if you weren't a strong, determined woman. Draw on your inner strength, say no to helplessness, and choose to be your own source of change again.

As I embarked on my own journey of discovery, I had a few of those 'WOW!' moments of experiencing something for the first time. The moments came in various forms; from a first yoga class, guided by the sweet, soothing voice of a senior teacher, to learning about the connection between my heels and the base of my skull through massage, to enjoying acupressure massages that transported me to a state of calmness beyond words. Every time, the way I related to myself changed almost immediately and propelled me to become more aware of how my body and mind work together.

Perhaps you have had similar experiences but have forgotten the peace they brought. Or, maybe, you have already begun to implement certain self-care practices, but need new or more effective tools to remind you of the vigour of feeling well-rested. After all, when we become mothers, every ounce of our attention shifts to those little love bundles, and we grossly neglect ourselves somewhere in between late-night wake-up cries, mum brains, and trying to keep our houses in order. Whatever your current situation, I believe you will find the techniques in the coming chapters easy and fun to practise.

At the beginning of my journey, I had no idea why it felt oh-so-delicious to experience vibrance and tranquillity at the same time. It was weird— a paradox. But I unashamedly craved more and could not get enough. These days, I draw on everything I've learned to help other mums understand the importance of self-care.

Self-care is fluid. It means different things to different people. I have experienced changes in my own approach to self-care over the years and have found that while indulging in luscious massages or attending yoga classes provide excellent nourishment, self-care entails so, so much more.

Rest Bite Takeaway

You are the cornerstone of your family, so it's not only your right to practise self-care, it's your responsibility. Stop treating self-care as an optional luxury you cannot afford because it's the one thing you *need* if you want yourself and your family to thrive.

What Is Self-Care?

Self-care begins with a realisation. For me, it was my uneasiness and reluctance to accept that my exhaustion and discomfort were 'just life'. Your story may look different. You might have woken up one morning and realised life is short and you need to make the most of your time. Maybe you feel guilty because you forgot the details of what was supposed to be a precious memory with your partner or child. Whatever it is that inspired you to look for answers, such as buying this book, that was your first step to self-care. The second but most important component of self-care is making a choice not to settle for whatever you feel restless about. Third, it is a practice that entails making time for yourself to take care of your needs—whatever they may be.

How To Make Self-Care A Part Of Your Life

The guidelines I'll share below entail many aspects of your life as a parent. You'll learn what self-care means for both you and your child and how you can use it to cultivate stronger, more meaningful relationships within your household. Later, in the remaining chapters, you'll delve deeper into relaxation techniques such as mindfulness and taking care of your body.

See Self-Care As A Way Of Life, Not A Random Activity

When you make self-care the priority it deserves to be in your life, interesting things happen. At first, you may experience slight pangs of guilt. You may feel like you're taking away something from your child.

What if he needs you while you're taking care of yourself?

It's a valid concern for a mother. However, by not taking care of yourself, you're really depriving yourself and your child of meaningful interactions. Think about it:

How many times have you been mentally far, far away, even though you were physically present?

How many times have you had bursts of anger at simple incidents, only to ask yourself how you could lose it over something so trivial?

How many days have you wished away because you were exhausted?

When you respond in a way you, nor your partner, nor your child expects, it doesn't make you a bad person or mother. It makes you human—one in need of some serious self-love and relaxation.

> ### Rest Bite Takeaway
>
> The best thing you can do is be open about what you're going through. Talk with your partner and with family and friends you trust. Your mother, aunts, and friends with children can relate to you and perhaps offer to babysit for a short while. Say yes! Grab those rare opportunities and use them to practise self-care.

Your child, however small, has an amazing learning capacity, and emotional intelligence is part of her early development. Around 8 months old, your baby will become aware of other people's feelings, especially yours, since she spends most of her time with you. Now is the best time to bring self-care into your life. Your baby will learn that little bits of time away from you is OK (you'll be OK, too, I promise), and she'll grow up understanding that everyone has needs—even her mama. She'll become a compassionate child and respect boundaries. Whether your love bundle is still a baby, toddler, or an older child, it's never too late to restructure your family's way of life to encourage self-care for everyone. By taking care of your own needs, you and your partner will be happier parents with higher energy levels to enjoy your child's most zestful days.

Self-Care Rituals You Can Start Implementing Today

When people hear 'self-care', scenes of manicures, pedicures, hours of massage sessions, and sips of champagne pop into their heads. While those sound idyllic, it's not possible for us mums. You'll be surprised how simple changes in your daily life can clear your head and make you feel like you've regained control. That said, I encourage you to explore and implement the restorative methods you'll learn in Chapters 4 to 7, because those methods are incredibly powerful and will take you on a journey of self-discovery like you've never experienced before.

In the meantime, the following guidelines will work wonders.

Understand Yourself

As strange as it sounds, few people know themselves these days. Most are so caught up in their routines that they function like robots. They rarely give thought to what triggers them to react in certain ways or even to what they enjoy.

The evidence of a lack of self-knowledge becomes apparent in conversations with others, where you may hear friends and even acquaintances describe you in ways you have never considered.

If you spend time with a journal, pen, and your own thoughts for as little as 5 minutes a day, you can learn (or rediscover) important things about yourself, like:

- What kind of temperament do you have?
- What are your personal limits?
- What are you passionate about?
- What activities do you love?
- What is the one thing you could do before bed to help you sleep better?

When you understand yourself, you can identify triggers that upset you and find ways to either navigate around those triggers or teach yourself to react differently when they emerge. Also, by exploring how you can make the best of your bedtime routine, you'll discover that something quite simple can make a massive difference in the quality of your sleep. For example, you might find that reading helps your brain shut down or that having a conversation with your partner before you turn the lights off alleviates stress.

Feed Your Soul

Every human wants meaning in life. For some, the source of meaning lies in religion; for others, it's simply a matter of connecting with nature and other people. No matter how busy you are, take some time to connect with your spiritual side—your body and mind will reward you for it.

You could do a quick prayer, go to a park with your baby, listen to motivational podcasts, or have a deep conversation with someone you look up to.

Meditation is one of the best ways you can feed your soul. In Chapter 7, I'll teach you how to practise restorative yoga poses.

Leave Work At The Workplace

Granted, we know this is easier said than done. Many mums work from home now, and working hours do not fit in that 9–5 box anymore.

Whether you have a traditional job or you work from home, this suggestion remains the same. As a dynamic woman, you take on many different roles. You're a wife, daughter, aunt, mentor, friend, and professional. For some reason, we're all efficient at switching roles without having one interfere with the other—except for work. Work stalks us; it demands to be a part of whatever we are supposed to do after work hours, and it leaves us feeling stressed over this and that task the moment we sign off.

Freeing yourself from overwhelming thoughts and concentrating on the present moment is a part of practising mindfulness, which we'll talk about in detail in Chapter 4. For now, though, it's within your reach to refuse work in your personal space. Find a way to let your mind transition from 'working mode' to 'personal mode' before you engage in the activities you would normally do after work. What works for you may not work for me, and vice versa.

Try different methods, like drinking a cup of tea, going for a brisk walk, or listening to your favourite feel-good song. Choosing to leave work where it belongs is empowering and a wonderful way to lower your stress levels.

Distinguish Between Needs And Wants; Then Say 'No'

This practice may be more applicable to mums with toddlers and older children since it is difficult to discern whether babies need or want attention in most cases.

As parents, it's natural to put our children's needs before our own. Without clear boundaries, they may take advantage to get what they want. Soon, you may find yourself at your child's beck and call for everything by mistaking desires for needs.

By lovingly asserting that you can't or don't want to do something right away when you know your child is expressing a desire instead of a need, you are practising self-care and teaching your child to be sensitive to others' needs. When doing this, communicate clearly by telling him/her, 'I hear you calling, but I'm busy with this thing. Let me finish, then I'll be with you' or, 'I know you want a snack. I would like one too, but it's almost time for dinner, and our appetites will be spoiled if we eat snacks now. We can eat some tomorrow'.

Toddlers, especially, are in the process of learning to deal with their emotions. If you have one, prepare yourself for tantrums when practising this technique. Parenting styles differ, so I will not advise you on how to deal with those tantrums. However, I would like to point out that sometimes it's best to let your little one go through his motions. He/she needs to vent to get rid of frustrations, just like adults need it. Of course, he'll/she'll learn to deal with frustrations in more constructive and socially acceptable ways as he grows and learns to understand his emotions and how they affect him/her.

Saying 'no' is difficult when you know it can upset your love bundle. On the other hand, if used in a positive way and seen as a learning tool, this practice can help you raise a person who will be emotionally secure and considerate of those she interacts with. Always keep in mind you are preparing your child for adulthood and helping her form habits that will likely accompany her for the rest of her life.

Rest Bite Takeaway

It's time to unleash your inner Rest Rebel. Choose at least 2 of the self-care rituals in this section to start practising today.

Knowledge is power: You hear it all the time, but knowledge is not power. It's only potential power. It only becomes power when we apply it and use it.

(Jim Kwik)

Other Useful Self-Care Methods

- Take frequent breaks during the day to keep your stress levels low.

- Eat nutritious food and snacks (part of knowing yourself is understanding how your body reacts to food).

- Make changes in areas of your life that aren't contributing to your happiness.

- Create a safe, enclosed environment where your baby or toddler can explore and play.

- Engage in positive inner talk, and don't be too harsh on yourself when you make mistakes.

How To Make Self-Care A Part Of Your Life

Habits contribute to how humans behave and interact with the world. So, the most effective way to integrate self-care into your life is by treating it as a new, healthy habit. However, as you know, habits are tricky to form. If we don't practise them frequently, or if we neglect them, they'll abandon us.

> In essence, if we want to direct our lives, we must take control of our consistent actions. It's not what we do once in a while that shapes our lives, but what we do consistently.
>
> (Tony Robbins)

Here are the steps I follow whenever I want to form new habits.

Step 1

Start with the self-care ritual that resonates with you the most. That way, it will feel like less effort to practise. With all your responsibilities, the last thing you need is to do something burdensome.

Step 2

Take your time to make the self-care ritual a part of your life. The goal is not to see how long you can practise it, but to practise it daily. If you can dedicate 2 minutes a day to your new ritual, then give it your all in those 2 minutes. Increase the time you spend practising your ritual only when you're ready—whether it takes a month, or 6, doesn't matter.

Step 3

Add another ritual that resonates with you when you're confident the first one has become second nature, and repeat the above process.

Rest Bite Takeaway

The kindest thing you can do for yourself while forming self-care habits is to be patient and consistent in your efforts. There is no reason to put pressure on yourself. You're not doing this for anyone but yourself. However, in choosing to focus a little of your energy on yourself, you are laying the foundation to be more mentally and emotionally available to your family, which will contribute to a happier, fulfilled household.

Use the space below to write down any thoughts or feelings you are experiencing right now. Be sure to add a date so you can see how much you've grown as a person when you come across this page in the future.

_____
_____
_____
_____
_____
_____
_____
_____
_____
_____
_____
_____
_____
_____
_____
_____
_____
_____

Chapter 4
Mind To The Rescue

Meditation and mindfulness are no longer foreign concepts. Both have become buzzwords, and many people—if not most—have heard that meditation is good for them. Everyone knows at least one friend who is glued to their yoga mat, always on the lookout for an opportunity to take a meditation break. For all its buzz, though, not everyone knows how meditation is supposed to be good for them. Some believe its reported effects are 'all in the mind', so they brush it off as the latest fad. Well, they're absolutely right about the first part!

The benefits of meditation are no fad, though. In fact, ample studies have been done on this fascinating field to prove its effectiveness. From reducing stress to improving your sleep quality, meditation has got you covered. In this chapter, you'll look at the science behind meditation, peek into its history, and then learn simple exercises you can practise before you move on to the next chapter.

I was lucky enough to have discovered meditation before I had my child. Back then, I had all the time in the world to engross myself in the intricacies of this brain-changing, patience-developing, compassion-promoting practice. When I welcomed my son into the world, all the time spent learning and applying meditation became mere memories. Some days, it felt as if I had dreamed it all.

Earlier, I told you that the only thing you can do is adapt to your new way of life. Of course, I had to do the same. Determined, I developed new-mum-friendly meditation exercises to keep my sanity and boost my happiness on those overwhelming days.

> With every breath, the old moment is lost; a new moment arrives. We exhale and we let go of the old moment. It is lost to us. In doing so, we let go of the person we used to be. We inhale and breathe in the moment that is becoming. In doing so, we welcome the person we are becoming. We repeat the process. This is meditation. This is renewal. This is life.
>
> (Lama Surya Das)

The History And Science Behind Meditation And Mindfulness

Meditation is an ancient practice and comes in many forms. Whatever the technique, the initial goal is always the same: to put yourself in a mental and emotional state of calm. Mindfulness is the practice of directing all your thoughts and energy to the present moment so you can be fully aware of what you're thinking, doing, and feeling right now. Combined, these 2 practices become 'mindfulness meditation', a powerful self-care technique that can make your life easier and contribute to your health and happiness. With constant practise, its effects will spill into how you interact with people and challenges—something every mother who has unintentionally lost her cool with her love bundle will appreciate.

The History

Many historical studies have looked into the origins of meditation without much success in pinpointing a year or even a culture in which it started. Despite this, meditative-like practices have been recorded for thousands of years, with the earliest written records coming from the Hindu and Buddhist cultures of India and the Taoist culture of China. No one can identify any record as the official starting point, but scholars agree that the above cultures were instrumental in spreading meditation to the rest of the world.

During the 1700s, Eastern philosophical texts with references to meditation made their way into the Western world and were translated into European languages. The West may have been introduced to meditation at an earlier date, but this period is typically accepted as the starting point. Despite its relatively early introduction, meditation remained a philosophical topic and received little to no interest from the public. This would all change in the early 20th century, when Hindu monk and philosopher, Swami Vivekananda, delivered a presentation on Eastern spirituality at the Parliament of Religions in Chicago. His presentation led to more and more Westerners craving knowledge about Eastern practices. However, what was considered deeply spiritual in the East, would take on a new character in the West.

In the West, meditation was revered for its mental and physical health benefits, so much so that its popularity invited scientific enquiry as early as the 1960s and 1970s. As study after study confirmed what people who had been practising meditation promoted, the scientific community and clinicians promoted its use for anyone—not just those who sought enlightenment.

The year 1979 marked a turning point for the use of meditation as a respected method to treat stress-related conditions. Jon Kabat-Zinn opened the Stress Reduction Clinic and used a program he called Mindfulness Based

Stress Reduction (MBSR) to treat patients. His work would lay the foundation for subsequent studies about the health benefits of meditation, especially with regard to mental well-being.

Despite its well-researched health benefits, meditation's popularity only peaked among the masses during the early 1990s. Since then, it has been growing strong and continues to change lives every day. Jon Kabat-Zinn's 1979 program, together with the work of Williams, Teasdale, and Siegel (1995)—who used Kabat-Zinn's program to develop Mindfulness-Based Cognitive Therapy (MBCT)—continues to be used in meditation research. There are now hundreds of proven mindfulness-based programs offered around the world, with more being developed every year.

If you are new to meditation, it is natural to wonder how it can help you and why, as a busy mother, you should even give it a try. So, before I introduce the exercises, I'd like to tell you about how meditation can impact various aspects of your life.

The Science

In the last 10 years, the field of neuro-imaging has been inves-tigating how meditation and mindfulness affect the brains of people with long-term meditation experience. Studies have consistently shown that engaging in these practices can change the structure of your brain, including changes in brain tissue thickness, increased neurons, and increased density in grey matter and white matter.

The regions where changes were noted are responsible for emotional and awareness-related functions, such as self-control, reactions, attention, and awareness of touch and pain.

A Harvard Medical School neuroscientist, Sara Lazar, discovered that people aged between 40—50, who had been meditating for a long time, had a similar density of grey matter in their frontal cortices as younger people (into their 30s). This is significant, as that part of the brain tends to decrease with age, which contributes to age-related memory loss. However, Sara Lazar's study showed that meditation can slow and even prevent this from happening.

Later, she wanted to see the effects of meditation on the brains of people who were unfamiliar with meditation. She sent them for a mindfulness-based stress reduction training program and had them practise other mindfulness exercises. Her study showed promising results and proved the effectiveness of mindfulness and meditation on the brain, even within a short period for those who had not meditated before.

Here is a summary of what the study found:

The region that controls your emotions, learning capacity, and memory, and the region responsible for empathy and compassion can increase. At the same time, the region that controls your responses to threatening or stressful situations can decrease. These structural changes translate into an increased capacity to better assess situations, control your emotions, and be less reactive when things go wrong—as they so often do when you're raising the next generation.

The Important Connection Between Breathing And Feeling In Control

When you pay attention to and pace your breathing, regions of your brain responsible for emotions, attention, and breathing activate. These are the same regions that undergo structural changes when you practise mindfulness meditation over time. This makes sense when you consider that being aware of how you inhale and exhale is a form of mindfulness, or living in the moment.

Many people still believe that breathing is exclusively linked to the brainstem and purely a physiological function for survival. However, A new study in the Journal of Neurophysiology discovered that when you pace your breathing, your body not only uses brainstem neural networks, but also those linked to awareness, attention, and emotion.

It also showed that quick breathing can increase feelings of fear, anger, and anxiety. Typically, when something unexpected happens, it's all too easy to become irritable, scared, or angry. In turn, your breathing also becomes more rapid, fuelling those feelings and pumping stress hormones throughout your body.

Rest Bite Takeaway

The next time you feel like you just might lose it, take the deepest breath you can muster, hold it in for 2 to 3 seconds, and release it slowly. Repeat this 3 to 4 times, and pay attention to how your mind instantly starts to relax instead of working against you with negative thoughts.

As with studies on meditation and mindfulness, science has now caught up with ancient wisdom. Controlled breathing exercises do indeed help you manage your mood and thoughts, thereby contributing to how you respond to stress.

Clinically Proven Benefits: How Meditation Can Impact Various Aspects Of Your Life

As a fellow mum who has gone through the above scenario and experienced first-hand how meditation has helped me be less reactive to stressful situations, I honestly believe it is a superpower. The women I have helped in my practice have all praised meditation as one of the best things they could have learned in their life's journeys. With simple, consistent meditative practices, the following benefits await you.

Reunite With Your Long-Lost Friend: Sleep

Studies on the effects of mindfulness on people's ability to sleep have found that it not only improves insomnia, but also improves sleep quality for those who do not suffer from sleep disorders.

Because mindfulness meditation brings about a relaxed state of mind, it's perfect for helping you fall asleep after you have put your baby to bed. With practice, you can teach your mind to become 'quiet' before bedtime, which means racing thoughts cannot prevent your mind from shutting down. Although studies are ongoing, researchers already suggest that meditation causes long-term changes in the brain, as they have found that experienced meditators enjoy improved REM and slow-wave sleep and experience fewer sleep interruptions during the night.

Meditation relaxes your body, too, by slowing down your breathing and heart rate. When that happens, it produces less cortisol, which also contributes to preparing you for a peaceful night's sleep (or at least high-quality, uninterrupted sleep until your baby calls for you).

Experience Less Anxiety And Enjoy Lower Stress Levels

On average, women experience more anxiety in various aspects of life than men; and as mothers, our minds are constantly weighed down with concerns over our children's safety and happiness, on top of worrying about our families' well-being, our financial situations, and other pressing matters. Left unchecked, our worries can become so excessive that they might lead to chronic stress and depression.

Meditation has the power to take your mind off worrisome thoughts and to help you keep them under control, which translates into less stressful days. Studies show a link between meditation and decreased anxiety, especially in people who have high levels of it and those who suffer from anxiety disorders.

If you have ever wondered if there is anything you can do to calm your mind just a little—even for a moment—you now have the answer. Science has given all mums the perfect 'excuse' to practise some well-deserved self-care in the form of meditation. When I say 'excuse', I don't mean to refer to an excuse you have to make to someone else to justify taking a break. Instead, it's the excuse (permission, if you will) you can give yourself without feeling guilty.

> ### Rest Bite Takeaway
>
> The mothers I have worked with have varied and unique stories. Some have partners while others are single parents. Whatever the case, there is one undeniable truth: **Mum is the most important person in your baby's life.**

Stress is destructive and can damage bodies, minds, and relationships if left unchecked. Meditation has been studied extensively in relation to stress management, and the science confirms what people from thousands of years ago already knew: If you want to live with less stress, just make meditation a part of your life. Mindfulness meditation, especially, is very effective. It creates an internal environment of relaxation, giving your body the resources it needs to use oxygen to the maximum, reduce stress hormones, improve your immunity, and even help your mind age slower.

If you meditate often, you'll perceive daily challenges as less stressful, you'll cope better with unexpected events, and you'll be able to recover from challenging situations with more ease.

Increase Your Attentiveness And Lengthen Your Attention Span

One of the weirdest and most embarrassing experiences for any new mum is when you realise something just happened, but you have no idea what it was. Being physically present and mentally absent is part of mummy brain (also known as mum's brain), a popular phrase that refers to the changes in women's' cognitive functioning when they have children. Typical characteristics of these changes include forgetfulness, hitting blanks, or talking about one thing while you mean to refer to another. Although the phrase sounds humorous and causes eyebrow-raising worthy behaviour, its realities are no laughing matter—at least not during the moment.

With meditation in your life, you can effectively alleviate the symptoms associated with mummy's brain. Studies prove that even in the short term, and with little to no prior experience in its practise, meditation improves the brain's ability to focus. If you've been plagued with not knowing where you had put your car keys or mobile phone seconds ago, you'll appreciate how effective mindfulness training can be. Also, you'll experience fewer moments where you have to ask someone to repeat her comment or question because your mind was simply not 'there'.

The length of time you can concentrate on tasks can also improve when you meditate often. Some researchers stated from their studies that meditation had altered patterns in their study group's brains that contributed to poor attention spans, scattered minds, and anxiety, effectively reversing and rewiring existing patterns into ones that contributed to longer attention spans and less worrying. And another promising study showed practising meditation for around 13 minutes a day improved people's memory and ability to focus daily in just eight weeks.

There you have it—science is on busy mums' sides!

Improve Your Emotional Well-Being And Self-Awareness

Every day, information bombards us. From the moment we wake to the moment we go to sleep, our minds absorb what we hear, see, smell, touch, and taste. Apart from our own problems, we hear, deal with, and try to help with the problems of our close friends and family members. And, of course, we act as our children's emotional guardians and try to shield them from the not-so-pretty side of life.

In a world where intellectualisation rules, it's hard to pause and connect with our emotional sides. It's strange because, above all, humans are emotional beings. I believe this same emotional disconnectedness is a major contributor to discontentment, frustration, and a lack of self-awareness.

There's nothing like meditation to help you find yourself again. In fact, a 2012 study found that meditation had such a profound impact on people's outlook on life that it advised clinicians to be aware of its ability to reduce stress-related symptoms and that they should have conversations with their patients about meditation programs.

Meditation helps your mind make sense of all the information you're confronted with every day and gives you a fresh perspective on situations that may trigger stress. Further, it helps you build skills to manage emotional overload, helps you build patience and resilience, boosts your creativity, and helps you to minimise negative reactions to stressful events.

With improved emotional well-being, you naturally become more aware of yourself and how you interact with others. Psychology talks of self-awareness as the ability to evaluate yourself with relative objectivity.

The ability to do this has advantages, like:

- you can become more sensitive to other people's challenges and develop more compassion and kindness;
- your self-esteem can improve, giving you more confidence in your mothering abilities and helping you not doubt yourself; you can practise more self-control in challenging situations; it can improve your communication skills;

- it can also help you make better decisions in various aspects, like finances, work, and family life.

Other Ways In Which You Can Benefit From Practising Meditation

- Meditation brings about physical benefits, like less pain, lower blood pressure, and an improved immune system.

- It helps alleviate the unique and varied challenges we ladies face before and during our menstrual cycles.

- Meditation can improve mental discipline for people who suffer from addictions.

- It helps keep the mind young by slowing age-related memory loss.

The best thing about meditation is that you can enjoy all its benefits without investing in expensive training programs or having to leave home to practise it. Above all, it does not demand hours and hours of your time to be effective. With 5 to 10 minutes of consistent, daily practice, the way you experience life can change 180 degrees.

Meditation is for mums what eyesight is for pilots. It allows us to see where we're headed, respond to conditions in our environment, and make adjustments when necessary.

(Amber Trueblood)

Simple, Effective, Busy-Mum Proof Meditation Exercises

The following exercises will introduce you to practising mindfulness. Even if you are familiar with mindfulness techniques, I encourage you to try the ones below to expand the toolset you already have.

The goal is simple: to ground yourself in the present moment and calm your anxious mind in moments of overwhelm. That said, by making this a daily habit for as little as 5 minutes, you'll soon experience a shift in the way you handle stressful situations. In time, your perception will change from, 'I don't know how to handle this', to, 'It's not that bad; what can I do to solve it?'

If you have time right now, do the following exercises as you read.

Experience The Breath

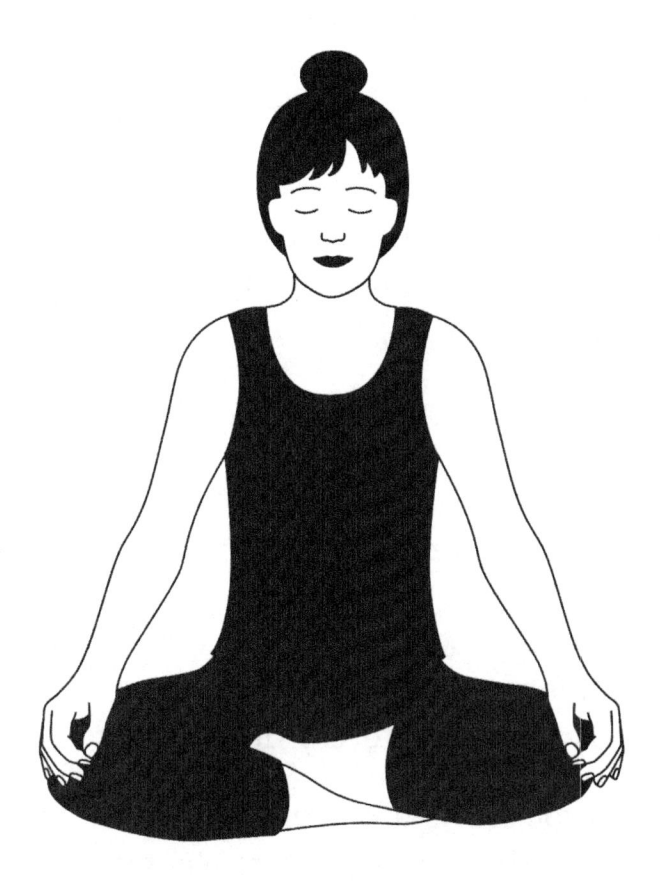

For this technique, you need to sit in a comfortable position. It's important that it's an easy position where you can sit straight and also where there are no distractions. You could use a chair or sit on the floor with crossed legs while supporting your spine with a cushion or bolster.

When you feel ready, close your eyes to help your mind concentrate on your body only.

Now focus on the rhythm, depth, and flow of your breathing. Observe the length of your breaths, but don't change anything about it. Be aware of the quality of the breath as it moves through you. Try to feel those tiny details:

- How does it feel at the tip of your nose as you inhale and exhale? Do you notice a change in temperature as the air moves in and out?
- Listen to the difference between inhaling and exhaling.

Be aware of your thoughts. If your mind has wandered from paying attention only to your breathing, refocus. You will get distracted often in the beginning. The important thing is that you become aware of where your mind is and bring it back every single time.

Know when you are breathing in, and know when you are breathing out. Think of nothing else but your breathing; embody it.

Still focusing on your breathing, it's time to broaden your awareness ever so slightly.

Let the sounds around you into your mental space.

Next, move your fingers slowly.

Be aware of the movement and the sensation of touch.

When you're ready, gently open your eyes.

If you do this exercise regularly, your breathing can become an anchor. This will always bring your mind to the present moment whenever it starts to wander away from whatever you are busy with.

Another version of this exercise entails pausing for a few seconds between inhaling and exhaling. Try both to see what works best to keep your mind in the here and now.

Count Your Breaths

Again, get yourself seated in a comfortable position. You can use anything for support if you are sitting crossed-legged.

As before, close your eyes and focus on your breathing.

This time, you will use counting to help you pay attention to this moment without allowing your mind to wander. Start with the number 20, and count backwards in your mind, like this:

- 'I am breathing in, 20.'
- 'I am breathing out, 20.'
- 'I am breathing in, 19.'
- 'I am breathing out, 19.'

Continue counting like this until you reach number one. As you progress, always be aware of where your thoughts are. If they wander or if you become distracted, bring it back to count your current breath and start at 20 again.

Sometimes, you'll feel tempted to speed up the process, so you'll breathe faster. Focus on filling up your breaths and staying calm. That way, the fullness of your breath will dictate the pace at which you count.

If thoughts slip in but don't distract you, it's OK to continue with the count. Just continue focusing on your breathing. You can repeat this exercise a few times, or start counting backwards from a higher number, like 50.

To end the exercise, follow the same steps as you did with the 'experience the breath' exercise.

Alternate Nostril Breathing

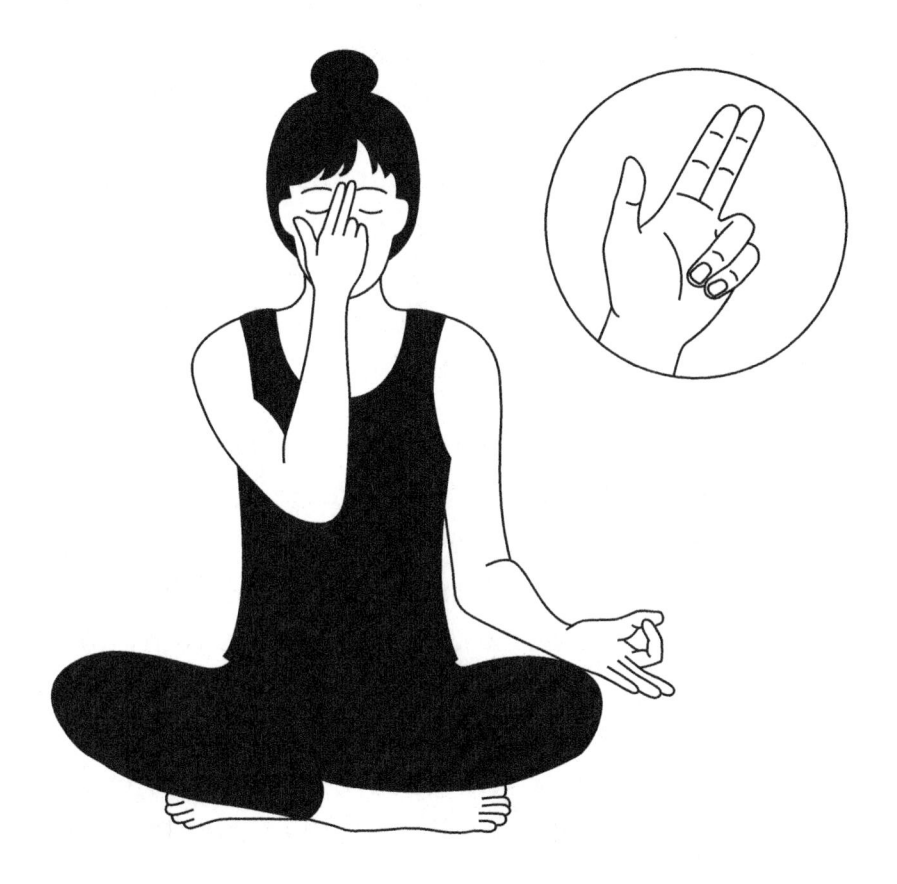

This is an exercise in breath control. It promotes balance in your body, increases your cognitive function, and helps you sleep better with regular practice. In time, you'll respond much better to stressful situations, as this is a very calming and grounding method with the power to help you fight off anxiety. From a physiological perspective, this exercise strengthens your lung muscles and helps you breathe easier.

This breathing exercise is best practised in a quiet space where there are no distractions. Sit upright so your chest can move easily during the exercise. Also, keep your shoulders relaxed the entire time.

Bring your right hand up to your face and gently place your index and middle fingers between your eyebrows. Rest your left hand on your lap or make a hand gesture called mudra by joining the tips of your index finger and thumb. When you're comfortable, exhale all your breath.

Press your thumb against your right nostril and inhale through your left nostril only. Keep at it until you have taken a comfortable, full breath. Now press your index finger against your left nostril, remove your thumb from your right nostril, and exhale through the right nostril. Keeping the pressure on your left nostril, inhale a comfortable, full breath through your right nostril. Press your thumb against your right nostril, remove your index finger from your left nostril, and then exhale through your left nostril.

The above instructions will help you complete one alternate nostril breathing cycle. Try to complete 8 to 10 complete cycles in one sitting. Try to keep your inhales and exhales for the same period of time. For example, when inhaling, count 1, 2, 3, 4 and when exhaling, count 1, 2, 3, 4, or whatever count works best for you. As your lungs grow stronger, you'll be able to extend your exhale counts much further (for example, you might count to 4 for your inhales and to 8 for your exhales). You might experience some dizziness or nausea when trying this for the first few times. If that happens to you, reduce the lengths of time you inhale and exhale; if the discomfort persists, it's best to stop practising for that day.

If you have respiratory issues or suffer from unchecked high blood pressure, the alternate nostril breathing exercise is best practised under supervision or avoided.

Abdominal Breathing

This is also called belly breathing because the focus is on moving your belly or abdomen when you breathe instead of just your chest. If you look at your baby while he's sleeping, notice how his belly expands and contracts as he breathes. This is natural and the way you're supposed to do it, too.

However, because of stressful lifestyles, most adults have succumbed to shallow breathing and no longer know what it's like to do it the real and right way. Note that you're not really forcing your abdomen to do anything when you practise this technique because when you take deep breaths, your diaphragm (which is at the base of your lungs) pushes your belly out.

Find a quiet place to lie on your back. When you lie down, place one palm on your chest and the other on your abdomen. Now breathe normally for a few moments and observe the movement of your hands on your chest and belly. If your belly is barely moving or not moving at all, your breathing is shallow, and it needs to change. Going back to natural breathing will help your body receive more oxygen and give you that extra boost of energy you need.

Breathe in as much air as you can while concentrating on allowing your abdomen to swell. Hold the breath for 3 to 5 counts, and release it slowly. If your abdomen does not contract as you breathe out, encourage it with a little pressure from the palm resting on it. It may take a while for the natural rhythm to come back.

Repeat the deep breaths around 10–15 times, all while focusing on your abdomen's movement. This exercise is all about focusing on your body's natural rhythm. If you realise you're not aware of how your belly moves while doing the exercise, bring your mind back to the moment and start again. Deep breathing like this triggers your body's relaxation response, so you'll feel quite refreshed when you get up to continue with your day.

Walking Meditation

It's so easy to switch to autopilot when driving or walking. How many times have you gone from point A to point B and wondered how you got there?

Walking meditation is an exercise aimed at helping you be fully aware of your surroundings and what you're doing while walking. You can do this exercise inside your home, but it might be more fun when you go for a stroll with your baby in the park or just around the block.

As you walk at a natural pace, pay attention to the lifting and falling of each foot as they move you forward. Be aware of your legs' movements and also of how the rest of your body responds as you move.

As with the other exercises, if you notice you're not concentrating on your body anymore and that your thoughts have carried you somewhere else, guide your mind back to what you are doing now. To help your mind stay focused, have an internal conversation about what you are experiencing. How does it feel when your feet hit the ground? When you take a turn, tell yourself, 'Now I am going in this direction'.

Next, expand your awareness to take in the sounds, smells, and sights of your surroundings, but constantly keep your mind on the moment. Don't allow your awareness of the environment to let your thoughts wander.

As you near the end of your exercise, guide your thoughts back to your body. Only focus on your feet, muscles, and how your body moves. When you're ready, pause for a moment and take in a few deep breaths to end your meditative walk.

In time, the effects of the above exercises will increase your awareness in all aspects of your life. You'll learn to appreciate each moment as it is and have more precious memories to reflect on, as they'll no longer slip your mind.

You're Not Too Busy For This

Yes, there is a lot to do. And yes, your time is limited. That said, as a mother, it is your responsibility to set personal boundaries and feed your soul with rest and give your body and mind a chance to rejuvenate.

Even if it means accepting you'll get less done in a day and giving your inner critic a rest—who never feels like she's doing enough, anyway—I encourage you to make time for this. Meditation will teach you how to just be and allow things to just be.

Start with 5 minutes a day and then build it up to as long as your free time allows or as your family commitments allow.

However you start, the choice must be yours. I have said this before: people (us mums, especially) are often our own worst enemies. We know what's best for us, but we sabotage our own needs to the point of feeling miserable sometimes. From now on, be kinder to yourself and find creative ways to take rest breaks. Here are a few ideas:

- practise mindfulness instead of hanging out on social media and endlessly scrolling through posts and comments;

CHAPTER 4: MIND TO THE RESCUE 123

- get up 15 minutes earlier so you can take care of yourself before taking care of the rest of the household;

- do a quick meditation exercise while your partner is giving your baby a bath;

- do a breathing exercise while you are waiting in the restaurant for your meal;

- make time for yourself while your baby is napping; instead of doing household chores while someone else is taking your baby for a stroll, meditate for a few minutes;

- while you're hanging out with your sweetheart, pretending to watch his favourite sport (he won't notice!);

- make some me-time while your toddler is occupied with story or music time.

I've heard it said that every day you need half an hour of quiet time for yourself, unless you're incredibly busy and stressed, in which case you need an hour. I promise you, it is there. Fight tooth and nail to find time, to make it. It is our true wealth, this moment, this hour, this day.

(Anne Lamott)

Use the space below to write down any thoughts or feelings you are experiencing right now. Be sure to add a date so you can see how much you've grown as a person when you come across this page in the future.

_____
_____
_____
_____
_____
_____
_____
_____
_____
_____
_____
_____
_____
_____
_____
_____
_____
_____
_____

Chapter 5
The Power Of Touch

How many times has your hand found its way to the back of your neck today? It's a reflex you may not even be aware of, but when your hands move to caress aching body parts like your shoulders, neck, and temples, it's your subconscious mind thinking ahead. In fact, these quick self-massages play a crucial role in helping you stay sane, mum brain and all.

> In everything we've done, massage is significantly effective. There's not a single condition we've looked at that hasn't responded positively to massage. Massage works because it changes your whole physiology.
>
> (Tiffany Field, PhD.)

Forgotten Wisdom: Massage Therapy In Ancient Times

These days, getting a massage is no longer considered a mere luxury. It's a necessity for those who seek alternative healing because of its amazing health benefits. But let's be honest... who among us has the time (or funds) for regular massages while raising children, running households, or working full-time?

As a massage therapist, I understand all too well how much my clients would love to check in with me frequently, but family life always comes first. Having studied massage therapy in its originating countries, like India and Thailand, I learned that massage is not only an important preventative health measure but a way of life. It is so ingrained into those cultures that most family members know massage techniques to relieve each other's aches and pains. Better yet, they like to massage each other simply because it feels so good. Postnatal recovery rituals in the Thai, Indian, and Chinese cultures include the use of healing herbs, eating nourishing food, and gentle oil massages during the first 40 days after giving birth.

Did you notice how I said getting a massage these days is '*no longer* considered a mere luxury?' However, the funny thing is that massages, in all its forms, were never leisurely activities to start with. It, like so many other health practices, has been around for thousands of years as a way of treating ailments.

Over the millennia, the ancient practice of massage has gone from sacred and revered, to being associated with indulgence and pleasure, to being ignored by mainstream medical practitioners, to regaining its rightful place as an effective treatment to heal the body and relax the mind.

The earliest evidence that humans used massage to ease pain and heal injuries comes from India, Egypt, and China around 5,000 years ago. In China, knowledge from ancient doctors, Buddhists, Taoists, and martial arts practitioners have contributed to recognising the importance and effectiveness of massage therapy. Modern Chinese methods, such as acupuncture and acupressure, are deeply rooted in the philosophy that ailments come from an imbalance in the energy found in certain locations in your body, which are connected to your physiological systems. When those areas (also known as energy channels) get massaged, it promotes energy to flow better throughout your body so it can heal itself. In Chapter 6, I will introduce you to wonderful self-acupressure techniques.

Having learned about massage as a healing practice from the East, the Greeks introduced it to Western civilisation around the 8th century BCE. Massage therapy was especially popular among athletes, who used it to ensure their bodies were properly prepared for competitions. Greek physicians introduced the use of oils and herbs in combination with massage therapy, which led to women recognising its benefits as a beauty treatment. Hippocrates promoted massaged therapy, together with rest, healthy food, exercise, and fresh air to promote optimal health.

Anyone wishing to study medicine must master the art of massage.

(Hippocrates)

Massage therapy became a part of Roman culture during the 1st century, BCE. As Western culture evolved into the common era, the medical landscape changed with new scientific findings. In the 1600s, there was a resurgence of massage therapy among Western physicians, but there were few advances in the techniques used. During the early 1900s, the West seems to have gone through a period of rediscovery. More emphasis was placed on the importance of massage therapy, which played a crucial role in treating World War I soldiers' shell shock and nerve-related injuries. Even so, it remained a luxury reserved for the wealthy in the eyes of the public. From the 1970s, however, people started seeking out holistic, natural methods to stay healthy and treat illnesses, and this movement has been growing stronger since. Thanks to people's demands for alternative healthcare, massage therapy has regained its rightful place in society as a valid, effective method to maintain and treat mental and physical well-being.

While it's all well and good to understand the health benefits of massage, it doesn't take away a mother's endless responsibilities and lack of time. That's why I want to introduce you to the power available at your own fingertips. Self-massage is one of the most effective self-care methods you can use to enhance your sense of calm and well-being. It can stimulate your lymphatic system, strengthen your immune system, and optimise your body's ability to remove toxins. With that comes improved blood flow, nourished skin, improved digestion, and a soothed nervous system. Apart from that, self-massage will give you the opportunity to learn about how pressure affects different parts of your body and help you understand how to massage your partner or another family member when life takes its toll on them.

The Benefits Of Touch

While some of us enjoy the company of fellow humans more than others, one thing remains true: we are social beings who thrive when we can enjoy physical contact. In fact, touch is one of the very first things all babies learn to process. It is important for cognitive and behavioural development. If this form of nurturing is lacking or absent during infant and early childhood development, it may translate into social, emotional, and physical issues.

Studies show that when we cannot experience physical touch for some time, we start feeling lonely and dwell on negative thoughts. The same studies also show that physical contact makes us feel satisfied, comfortable, and secure.

Physical sensation (and lack thereof) and its effects have been a topic of study in Western science for at least 200 years. No wonder there are various terms to describe the same need. Phrases like 'touch starvation', 'touch deprivation', 'touch hunger', and 'affection deprivation' all refer to what people go through when they crave physical contact after a period of not being able to experience it.

The benefits of touch are not just psychological. When you perceive touch as sincere, whether it comes from your partner, a family member, a friend, or even a handshake from a stranger, your body responds positively. When touch receptors under the skin get stimulated, your blood pressure and cortisol levels decrease, lowering your stress levels. The reward centre of your central nervous system is responsible for processing most forms of touch you experience throughout the day, which is why hugs, reassuring hand squeezes, and comforting strokes contribute to feeling joyous and content.

Rest Bite Takeaway

Touch is especially powerful between those in intimate relationships. The next time you get a chance to hug your partner, don't treat it as a formality. Really lean into it, observe the sensation, and notice how much better it makes you feel. Touching (or being touched) by someone you trust enhances the 'love hormone', oxytocin.

How Engaging In Self-Massage Can Save The Day

The benefits of touch are not limited to being in physical contact with others. Sometimes, when you're alone at home with your baby, and you really need to feel better, all you have to do is give yourself a quick massage. This is about the closest thing to a 'quick fix' you can get.

Ease Your Aches And Pains

A regular self-massage routine will help you feel relief from those pesky pain points that spoil your days. Dull pain does not stop you from engaging in daily activities and meeting your responsibilities, but it does get irritating and can affect how you respond to potential conflict, no matter how minor it may be. And let's not forget those other aches that come out of nowhere when your baby gets picked up, especially your shoulders and back. By the way, if you recently gave birth, you are more at risk of injury due to hormonal changes that loosen your joints and ligaments. Self-massage can help relieve the aches and pains that come with bringing a new little person into the world.

Sleep Better

Combined with the right essential oils, self-massage induces a relaxed feeling and helps your brain calm down as bedtime approaches.

Boost Your Circulation And Release Toxins

With improved circulation, your muscles will enjoy more blood flow and receive more oxygen, leading to less stiffness. With increased blood flow through your arteries and muscles, toxins shouldn't get a chance to hang around and give bacteria a platform to cause illnesses.

Balance Your Emotions

A less tense body releases an abundance of feel-good hormones and thereby increases your emotional well-being. When you are emotionally balanced, your body is more resilient against stress-related physical issues. With practicing self-massage comes feelings of being calm and in control of situations, and you'll also avoid being reactive in hair raising situations.

Experience Less Anxiety And Stress

When your body has a healthy supply of feel-good hormones and you feel in control, stress hormones tend to stay away for longer and do not dampen your mood that easily. You also gain the perspective to realise that not every potential conflict situation is worth drama. You also learn to accept more things you have little control over and start focusing more energy on tasks, people, and activities that contribute to a happier life.

How To Protect Your Body During Your Self-Massage Rituals

Self-massage is generally a safe self-care ritual, but you should take precautions to avoid hurting your soft tissues accidentally. So, when you engage in self-massage, avoid the following areas:

- Bruised skin.
- If you had surgery recently or have a healing wound, avoid that area, varicose veins, open cuts.

Also, don't practise self-massage rituals under the following conditions unless you consult your doctor or a certified Ayurvedic practitioner for guidance on how to do it safely.

- If you have severe hypertension.

- If you have a high fever.
- If you have a cold or flu infection.
- If you are menstruating.
- If you are pregnant.
- It's best to check in with your doctor before you engage in self-massage if you suffer from any medical conditions.

Self-Massage Rituals To Enrich Your Life

The following self-massage rituals have been adapted from my own therapy practice for home use. The mums who have been following these methods for some time now all say this is by far the most effective, as well as their favourite, self-care technique.

Calming & Grounding Oil Self-Massage

This massage's effects are most powerful when you do it in the morning or evening. You'll need to set aside 5–10 minutes and have a ⅓ cup of your favourite light massage oil handy. If you don't have a favourite yet, try sweet almond oil or fractionated coconut oil. You'll enjoy the best results if you can do this self-massage every day, but you'll still experience amazing benefits from doing it just 2–3 times a week.

Sit on a towel in a dry, warm room for this self-care ritual. Starting with your hands, gradually massage the oil into your entire body. Pay special attention to your palms, each finger, and your knuckles. Move on to your arms with long strokes and circular movements around your joints.

Spend extra time tending to your wrists and elbows.

Next, massage your feet, and make sure you give the soles of your feet, each toe, the webbing between your toes, and the back of your heel extra love. Massage the oil into your legs. Make long strokes over the legs and circular movements on your knees; be sure to give your knees some extra attention, too.

Rest Bite Takeaway

Direct all your thoughts to this moment. Tell yourself which part of your body you are tending to. Think of the kind of motions you're making, and have total awareness of the sensation on your skin as your hands move about your body. Breathe deeply and immerse yourself in the relaxing, positive feelings this self-massage brings.

Next, move upward to the middle of your body. As you progress with the massage, add extra oil to your skin as needed. Massage over your chest and shoulders. Apply circular, clockwise motions under each side of your collarbone. Make firm and long strokes around the back of your neck and lower shoulders and massage into your armpits. From there, continue over and around your breasts. This massage will help you become more familiar with your body and enable you to detect any changes, especially in your breasts.

Move toward your abdomen, first focusing on the left side where your large intestine is located. Maintain a downward stroke and then change the direction upward as you move over to the right side of your abdomen. As you move into your stomach area, make a circle back to the left. Continue this motion a few times to stimulate your abdominal and pelvic muscles and to support the natural flow of your digestive system. As you reach your ribs, massage underneath them to stimulate your spleen, pancreas, and liver.

Now you can move over to your back, hips, lower back, and sacrum area.

When you're done with your body, you can round off the massage by moving on to your head and face. Use light finger pressure and circular movements all around your face. Start at the top, end with your ears, and then stroke down your neck. You can massage some of the oil into your hair and scalp. Gently tug your hair as you massage the oil into the roots.

If you have time, allow up to 10 minutes for your skin to absorb the oil after your massage. Afterwards, you can enjoy a warm bath or shower (not a hot one).

> Massage is not just a luxury. It's a way to a healthier, happier life.
>
> (Anonymous)

Whole Body Tapping

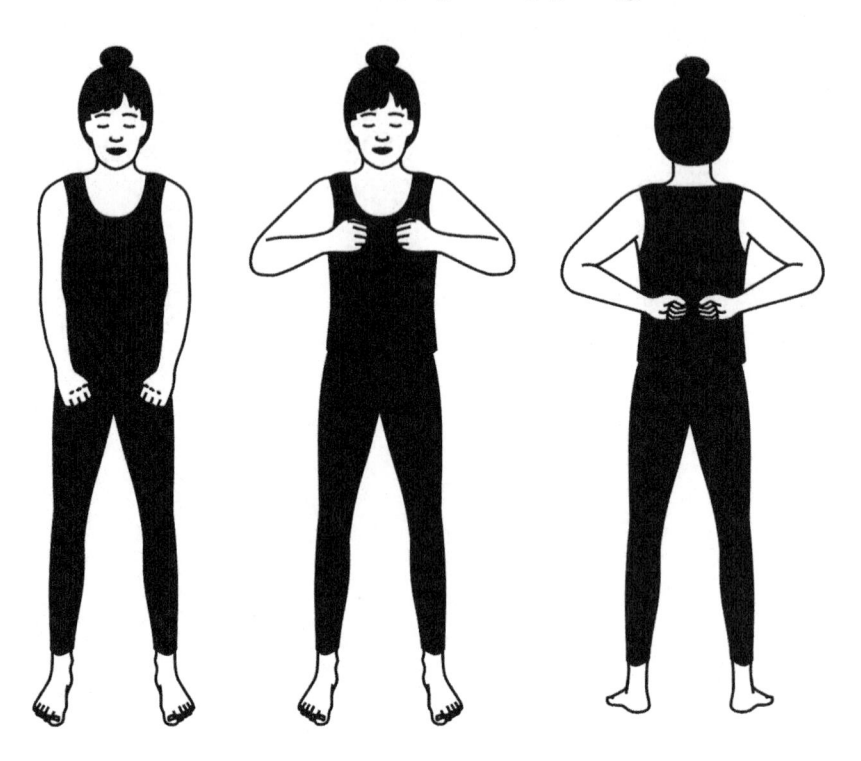

Body tapping is an ancient method that improves circulation and stimulates drainage of the lymphatic system, promoting the release of toxins. It's also a very effective method to stimulate the energy channels throughout your body. According to traditional Eastern medical practices, these energy channels may cause imbalances and diseases when blocked or depleted. Studies have been done on these energy channels in the West, and some suggest that they may indeed be linked to our bodies' central nervous systems.

This is my go-to self-care ritual on most days.

It does not require the use of oils, and you can do it fully clothed. The method I recommend has its origin in the Japanese practice of Shiatsu, where you can rely a series of stretches and your fingers to bring relief.

The aim of whole-body tapping is to create physical and energetic balance. It is a short and easy routine, but it has the power to revitalise your strained muscles, decrease stiffness, ease your tired mind, and uplift your spirit.

You'll need 10 minutes for this exercise. Keep a natural posture and breathe normally whenever you practise this technique. You can do this exercise standing or sitting, but unless you have mobility issues, I suggest you do it standing.

Overall Bounce And Body Tapping

To start, spread your feet shoulder-width apart and keep them parallel to each other. Bend your knees slightly and bounce up and down. This need not be a vigorous bounce, but you should definitely get the feeling that you're bouncing your body as opposed to just moving it up and down at a slow pace. Relax your arms and shoulders, back, and hip joints while you bounce. While bouncing, take a deep breath, roll your shoulders forward, backward, and up, and then exhale as you drop your shoulders again. Repeat this 5 times and then change direction, repeating the motion another 5 times in the opposite direction.

Now, twist your torso from side to side and allow your arms to swing naturally with the motion. As your torso swings to the left, let your right fist tap under your left collarbone and your left arm tap against the right side of your spine in the area where your kidneys are located. Synchronise your breathing with the movements: when your torso comes back to the centre, inhale, and when it twists to the sides, exhale.

As you move, keep your gaze straight ahead. Keep the motion up for 1 to 2 minutes, and let your body move freely. It might feel strange in the beginning, but the movements are quite natural, and you'll get into the flow the more you practise.

When you're ready to move on to the next technique, realign your body in the centre and stand completely still for 20–30 seconds. To make this a mindfulness exercise, try to notice any changes in your body while doing body tapping.

Head And Face Tapping And Massage

To continue with the exercise, bend your knees slightly, hip width distance apart. Now tap against your head with open palms or your fingertips. Cover the sides, front, and back of your head. When you're ready to stop, run your fingers through your hair and gently pull on it.

To tend to your face, place your fingers around the centre of your forehead and stroke outward toward your temples with little pressure. Repeat this movement 5 times.

Massage your temples with gentle, circular movements. Keep your elbows down, and your shoulders relaxed while doing this. Move down the sides of your face and follow your jawline. When you reach the jaw area, use your index finger and thumb to pinch all along your jaw.

Now massage your eyebrows, starting from the centre between them and applying pressure as you move outward; do this 5 times. Next, use your thumb to stroke from the top to the bottom of your nose to clear your sinuses and release possible nasal congestion. Repeat this action 5 times, too.

Neck Tapping And Massage

Now place your right palm against the left side of your neck and massage firmly with a squeezing motion. Place your left palm against the right side of your neck and repeat the same process. Now place both hands behind your upper neck and move to the base of your skull. Apply pressure with both thumbs at the base of your skull and move along to the back of your ears, where you feel the protruding bones of your skull. Switch to your fingers and continue to massage the base of your skull in circular movements.

Shoulder And Arm Tapping

As you inhale, lift your shoulders and drop them in sync with your exhaling breath. Repeat this action at least 5 times, but you can go on longer if you'd like. Lift your right arm and tap against your left shoulder with a fist or open palm. Follow up with a massage by applying pressure in a circular motion over the shoulder. Stretch out your arm in front of you and tap from top to bottom on the inside of your arm with a fist or open palm. Tap the palm of your left hand a few times, turn your arm over, and tap upward, back to your shoulder. Now repeat the process 5 times, making sure you tap down the inner arm as you move down and the outer arm as you move up. After 5 repetitions, switch the tapping action over to your right arm (using your left fist or open palm).

With the 5th repetition of each arm, give your hand a thorough massage. Start in the middle by applying moderate pressure and moving toward the fingers in circular motions. Squeeze and massage each finger in turn.

When you're done, straighten your body again and relax for a moment.

> Almost everything will work again if you unplug it for a few minutes, including you.
>
> (Anne Lamott)

Chest, Abdomen, And Lower Back Tapping

Tap across your chest (staying above your breasts) with loose fists or open palms. Gradually work your way down to your abdomen. Once there, continue to tap, but switch to a clockwise, circular motion and keep it up for at least 1 minute. Now place one hand on top of the other and rub over your abdomen in the same circular motion for another minute.

Start tapping again, this time moving toward the sides of your abdomen and working your way around to your lower back, just under your kidneys. Do this for a minute to 2 minutes.

Now stop bouncing and lean forward. Place one hand on a knee to support your weight while you use the other hand to tap on and around your sacrum for about a minute.

Leg Tapping

From your sacrum area, move over to your hips and make your body a little straighter. Continue to tap, moving over to your buttocks. You can tap that area with fists or open palms. Move on by tapping down your back legs all the way to your heels (you can bend your knees to reach your heels). From your heels, move to your inner legs and continue tapping in an upward direction from your ankles to your groin area. From there, tap toward the outside (in line with your hips) and tap downward all along your outer legs and back up again.

Round it off by tapping on your abdomen for another minute. Afterwards, give your body a good shake, from your head to your shoulders, to your feet.

Feet Massage To End The Tapping Sequence

To finish this exercises, sit down and rest your right foot across your left thigh. Rotate your ankle in both directions to stimulate and loosen the joint. Start massaging your foot with your thumb and then move on to kneading it with both hands. After 1 minute, switch over to your left foot and repeat the process.

Once done, stand up straight with your feet shoulder-width apart. Close your eyes and imagine that a string runs from your sacrum, right through your spine, all the way to your head. Take mental notes of how you feel after the whole body tapping session, and try to recall how you felt before you did the tapping exercise. How do the two compare?

Rest Bite Takeaway

Keep a self-massage journal to see how your thoughts and feelings evolve as you engage more and more in these self-care rituals (whether it is the oil massage, whole-body tapping, or any other method you learn along the way). Write down your thoughts and feelings before you do a self-massage and again afterwards. Read the journal every 3 to 6 months to see how it impacts your emotional and physical well-being.

Before we continue... will you help a fellow mum find hope, too?

I contemplated about adding this part into the book, as the last thing I want is for you to feel like an annoying advert just popped up and ruined a good show.

Still, the message of this book is important for every new mum. So, my hope is that you'll receive this request with a warm heart and realise the impact your words can make on a mother out there who, undoubtedly, feels like she's drowning under exhaustion and stress.

By now, you're well aware of how crucial it is to prioritise your own self-care. You understand that putting yourself first in this sense means that you're really putting your little one first. You have also (hopefully) started implementing the strategies in the book and can probably feel the difference in your energy and confidence levels.

If you take a moment to share your honest opinion of how this book has improved your life, you'll be a guiding light, a beacon of hope, for other new mums. You'll be a friendly, relatable voice telling them they're not alone and that self-care isn't selfish at all. Better yet, you'll be the one guiding them to the answers they're so desperately looking for to take control of their lives again.

As you know, every new mum finds it tough in the beginning. But together, we can give each other the support we all need.

Please head over to Amazon.com and take five minutes to leave a review of Rest Bites—you really can change another mum's life for the better with your words.

Thank you so much for your support.

"Don't tell a mother she looks tired; she already knows that. Tell her she's doing a great job; she may not know that." (Stephanie Peltier)

Chapter 6
The Power Of Acupressure

In this chapter, you will explore the concept of energy channels further, with special emphasis on acupressure and how you can use this self-care method to allow energy to flow freely through your body. You will also learn about the history of acupressure and discover how applying pressure on specific parts of the body calms you down and makes you feel nurtured. Finally, I'll share easy self-acupressure techniques you can start using today.

What Is Acupressure?

Acupressure is an ancient massage technique with its origins in Chinese medicine. Most Eastern healing methods have the goal of encouraging the effortless flow of energy through the body, and acupressure is no different. Acupressure targets certain points along the energy channels that exist in the human body. Its goal is to enhance the flow of a specific energy called Qi (pronounced 'chi' or 'chee'). Qi basically means 'life force' or 'vital energy'. According to traditional Chinese medicine, Qi is crucial for physical, mental, and emotional well-being.

While you need not agree with the concept of Qi and energy channels, these Eastern healing methods carry scientific significance, and their impact on people's health is being studied by Western health practitioners more and more.

For example, it seems that applying pressure to the points targeted by acupressure releases endorphins, which are chemicals responsible for relieving pain. It is little surprise, then, that those who regularly receive acupressure treatments report reduced headaches, back pain, and body aches related to injuries.

Although research around acupressure and other Eastern healing methods are still new and inconclusive, those who use these self-care methods are willing to swear by the benefits they enjoy. Some of the most common benefits include nausea relief among pregnant women, better sleep, relaxation, faster healing of injuries, and improved digestion.

The Origins And History Of Acupressure And Acupuncture

Although no concrete evidence remains of the precise origin of acupressure, some historians speculate that the practice might be older than its more famous counterpart, acupuncture.

Acupressure and acupuncture target the same energy channels in your body, and both focus on the flow of Qi. However, acupuncture can only be performed by a certified practitioner, as it involves the insertion of needles as thin as a hair into specific areas of the body. These needles stimulate your energy channels to help your body regain balance. On the other hand, acupressure is all about applying pressure to those same areas of the body to stimulate those channels.

Both practices are thousands of years old and are equally effective. But for busy mums, acupressure is by far the most attractive option.

The general consensus is that acupressure and acupuncture started in China. Documents and artefacts confirm that around 2,000 years ago, the concept of energy channels and Qi were already well-known among Chinese Emperors and their ministers. One document, *The Yellow Emperor's Classic of Internal Medicine*, describes in detail a system of diagnosis and treatment that is nearly identical to what we know as acupuncture today. The foundation that practitioners use for acupuncture today had already been established during the Ming Dynasty, from 1368–1644.

As Western culture and medicine started playing more prominent roles in the East, the practice of acupressure, acupuncture, and other traditional Chinese medicines declined in popularity. In fact, by 1929, acupuncture and some traditional methods were banned altogether. It found its way back into public life some decades later and was subject to the forces of the cultural revolution. From here it has gradually regained status in the country of its origin as a core component of healthcare, with many hospitals now combining Western and Traditional Chinese approaches.

In Europe, acupressure and acupuncture were introduced by a European physician who witnessed them in Japan. The Japanese had learned it from the Chinese during the 6th century. Although these practices enjoyed some enthusiasm and interest throughout the earlier centuries of the common era, they did not gain momentum until the 1970s. Today, both acupressure and acupuncture are widely accepted practices and effective self-care rituals for people from all walks of life.

All Mums Can Do With A Healthy Amount Of Energy

You Yourself, as much as anybody in the entire universe, deserve your love and affection.

(Buddha)

Like I said earlier, you need not agree with the concepts of Qi and energy channels. However, I'm sure you'll agree with one thing: life requires an incredible energy reserve. (And being a mum requires even more than that!)

The amount of energy you have influences all aspects of your life, but— as you know all too well—its abundance or scarcity shows when it comes to vitality and wellness.

When you're low on energy, nothing works quite right. It causes exhaustion, frustration, a scattered mind, a lack of motivation, and a general sense of discouragement to face each day. On the other hand, when you have too much energy (you need not look further than a toddler for a good example), your mind becomes too busy with ideas, to-do lists, and hundreds of thoughts that keep you up at night.

Too little and too much energy have the same consequence: they prevent you from spending your days meaningfully and productively.

> ### Rest Bite Takeaway
>
> Taking care of yourself includes being aware of how you spend your days. Do you reach at least 2 of your goals (or tasks) on a daily basis? It's easy to say, 'I'm just too busy'. But, more often than not, we fail to get things done because of an imbalance in our lives. This chapter is all about teaching you how to help your body make the best of the energy reserves it has to restore balance in your life. That said, taking care of yourself is also a holistic approach. So, always practise mindfulness by being aware of how you spend your time. By simply being aware of how and where you lose time, you'll feel more motivated to implement balance restoring techniques to get you back on track.

According to traditional Chinese medicine, we all have a battery. This battery is influenced by two main sources:

- Qi inherited from our parents (pre-natal or pre-heaven Qi).

- Post-natal or post-heaven Qi.

This is influenced by how well we live our lives. Our choices of food, sleep quality, relationships, and emotional life. An appreciation and respect for nature's cycles and our own place within them. The Chinese call this Yangsheng—nourishment of life.

From a Western perspective, we may say Pre-natal Qi equates to our genetic heritage. Post-natal Qi lies within lifestyle and practices. In essence, the philosophy is that a balanced life, less stress, and consumption of high-quality foods equals more Qi. Looking at Western culture and health studies, we know that low stress and a healthy diet contribute to wellness and happiness. So, it's not hard to see the connection between the concept of healthy levels of Qi and practices that support it.

But for us mums, even lifestyle choices and better eating habits do not always do the trick. The good news is that 'low power mode' does not have to be a given in your life. In this chapter, I want to show you how to use the energy you already have to its full potential. The acupressure techniques I'll share will release and help energy flow through your body more easily. The acupressure points you'll learn can bring relief to issues like poor concentration or sleep, moodiness, anxiousness, and lack of energy. I would, however, like to point out that your current health condition will determine the speed and depth of impact. For example, if you have a chronic condition that contributes to your inability to sleep, you might not get results as soon as someone who does not suffer from the same or a similar condition. But don't let that discourage you. If there is one thing I can guarantee, it is that persistence and daily practise pays off in anything you do.

Understanding Acupressure Points

Your energy channels are located throughout the body. There are 12 ordinary channels, that are considered to be linked to your organs. Depending on the channels you target, the organs related to them will respond. There are also extraordinary channels, these influence the energy systems in a powerful way, and we use some points from these channels in our practices.

Along your channels are hundreds of acupressure points, also known as acupoints. When one of those points receives stimulation, energy starts to flow more freely and starts sending healing messages to the parts of the body associated with it. Acupressure is simply the act of applying pressure to any one of the acupoints located along your body's energy channels.

How To Locate Your Body's Acupoints

There are a few methods for locating acupoints, but we'll stick to the traditional method used by ancient Chinese practitioners, called the body inch or cun. To locate an acupoint, you have to make use of this measurement. 1 cun is equal to the width of your thumb's first joint (when viewed from the tip of the thumb). When seeing patients at my practice, I always use the anatomy of the person receiving the therapy for accurate measurement. This is because each of our bodies are unique when it comes to measurements. For example, 1 cun for you is not the same as 1 cun for your baby or your partner.

The diagram below illustrates other important acupressure units of measurement.

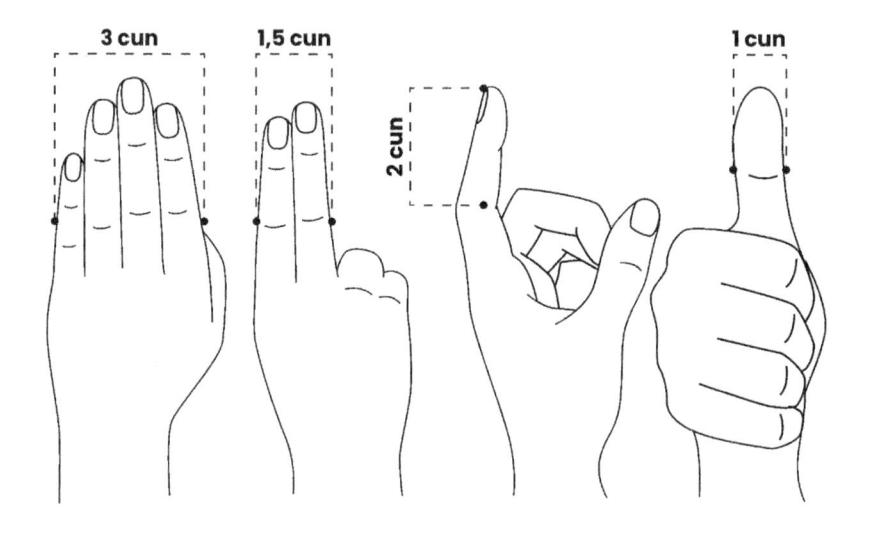

When to Avoid Acupressure As A Self-Care Method

Although acupressure is one of the safest ways to take care of yourself and does not pose any risk in most circumstances, you should consult your doctor before applying it if you suffer from acute or chronic health conditions.

Do not engage in acupressure under the following circumstances:

- if you have cancer in the vicinity of acupoints;
- have a bone condition, such as rheumatoid arthritis;
- have a spinal injury;
- if you have varicose veins in the vicinity of acupoints;
- if you are pregnant, as certain acupoints can induce contractions.

How To Practise Self-Acupressure

Unlike some of the techniques from the previous chapters, you do not need to block off time to practise this method. All you need to stimulate those potent acupoints is a free hand.

You can think of self-acupressure as an on-the-go self-care ritual. All you need is a deep breath, relaxed body, and awareness of which pressure points to activate. If you can, gently stretch your body before starting the acupressure by rolling your shoulders, stretching your body from side to side, and making any movements necessary to make your body feel as comfortable as possible. If you're at home or anywhere private, you can sit on a chair or crossed-legged on the floor, or you can lie down on a padded floor.

When applying pressure to your acupoints, use a firm but steady pressure, and increase it gradually. The sensation should be sensitive, but not painful. In essence, you're looking for a balance between pleasure and pain. You might also feel different sensations between different acupoints. If you hold on to an acupoint, it creates a calming effect; if you press down for 5 to 10 seconds, gently massaging in a circular motion, it stimulates the acupoint in a more active manner.

Rest Bite Points

I coined the following acupressure exercises *Rest Bite Points*, as I have identified them as the most potent to use in your self-care journey as a mother. Take your time to read through all of them before you decide on the one you'll try first.

Bubbling Spring Acupoint (Kidney 1)

This acupoint, also known as Kidney 1 or KI 1, helps to rejuvenate your spirit and your body's batteries (Kidneys). Considering its location, it's almost unthinkable that simply applying pressure to it can have such a profound effect on you. Some have described what happens as a surge of energy simply flooding through them.

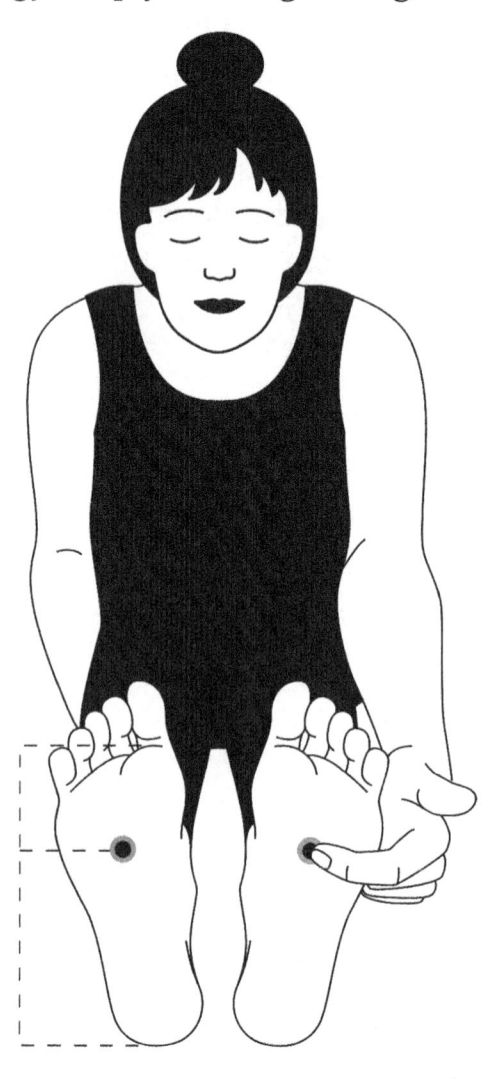

Location

KI1 lies in the middle of the balls of your feet. An easy way to find it is to curl your toes inwards and feel or look for the depression that forms. It's right underneath that depression.

How To Stimulate The Acupoint

Massage the point with your finger for at least 30 seconds. Alternate between your feet for 2 to 3 minutes.

Self-Reflection

After stimulating this acupoint, reflect on how you feel.

Date:_____

_____
_____
_____
_____
_____
_____
_____

Shenmai Acupoint (Bladder 62)

This acupoint can help you get a good night's rest. This point is better known as Bladder 62 or Bl 62 because it lies on the Bladder Channel. Apart from clearing your mind and inducing a restful state, practising acupressure on this point can also clear blocked energy and obstructions causing discomfort and pain in your bladder area.

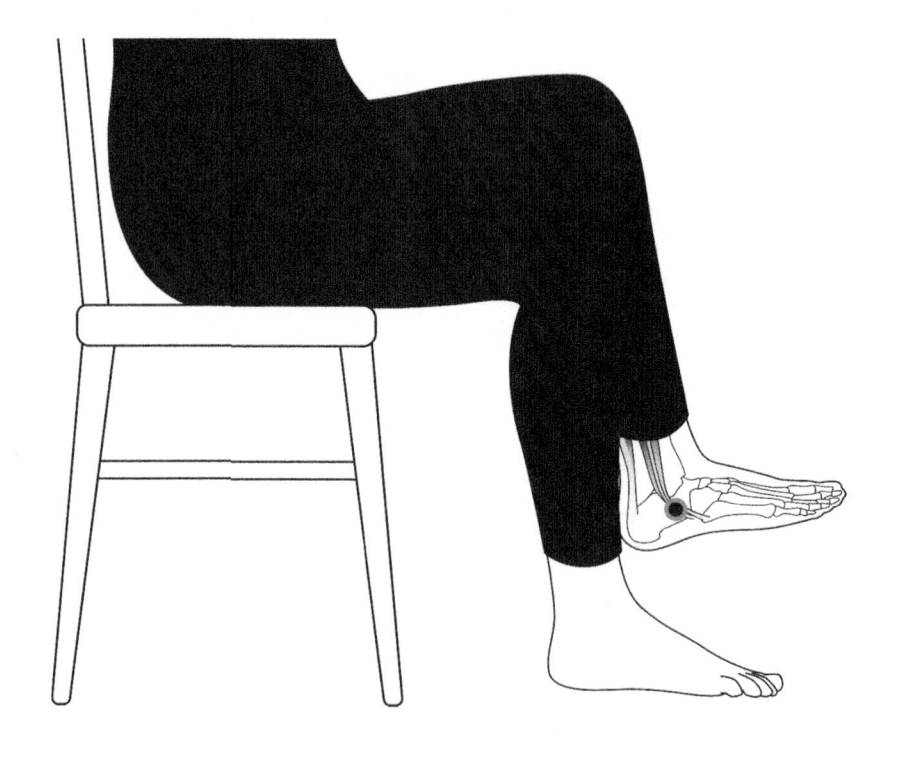

Location

Find the most prominent point on the outer ankle (lateral malleolus), directly below this prominence is a hollow, the acupoint lies within.

How To Stimulate The Acupoint

A few minutes before bedtime, get yourself in a comfortable position that will allow you access to your ankles. Apply pressure on the acupoints with 1 finger on each acupoint. Hold the pressure while taking deep breaths for around 3 minutes.

Self-Reflection

After stimulating this acupoint, reflect on how you feel.

Date:_____
_____
_____
_____
_____
_____
_____
_____
_____

Upper Sea Of Qi Acupoint (Conception Vessel 17)

The Sea of Tranquillity acupoint lies along the Conception Vessel channel, which runs along the front of your body's midline. Activating this point, also known as CV 17, can help you manage anxiety and stress and insomnia.

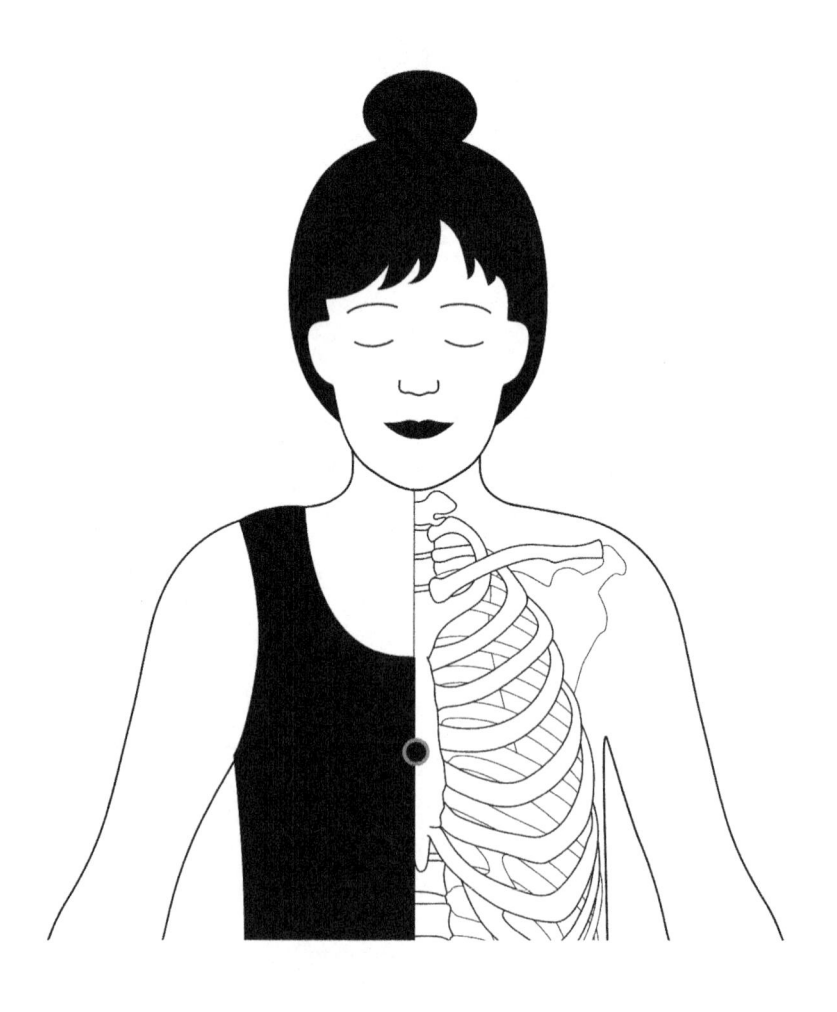

Location

C 17 sits on your breastbone, in the mid-line. Extend your 4 fingers and place them against your chest, with your pinkie finger at the base of your breastbone. Now let your index finger feel for a slight indentation in the area where it is resting. Once you feel the indent, you have found the right spot.

How To Stimulate The Acupoint

Make sure your spine is upright and straight, and take a few deep breaths. Using your thumb, apply gentle pressure to the acupoint for 2 to 3 minutes. Another way of stimulating this point is to sit up straight in bed and tap against the acupoint a few times before you sleep.

Self-Reflection

After stimulating this acupoint, reflect on how you feel.

Date:_____

_____
_____
_____
_____
_____

Shu Mansion Acupoint (Kidney 27)

Paired with acupoint C 17 above, Shu Mansion (also called Kidney 27 or K 27), brings powerful relief to feelings of depression, severe stress and anxiety, and worry. It is also effective in helping you breathe easier and clearing congestion.

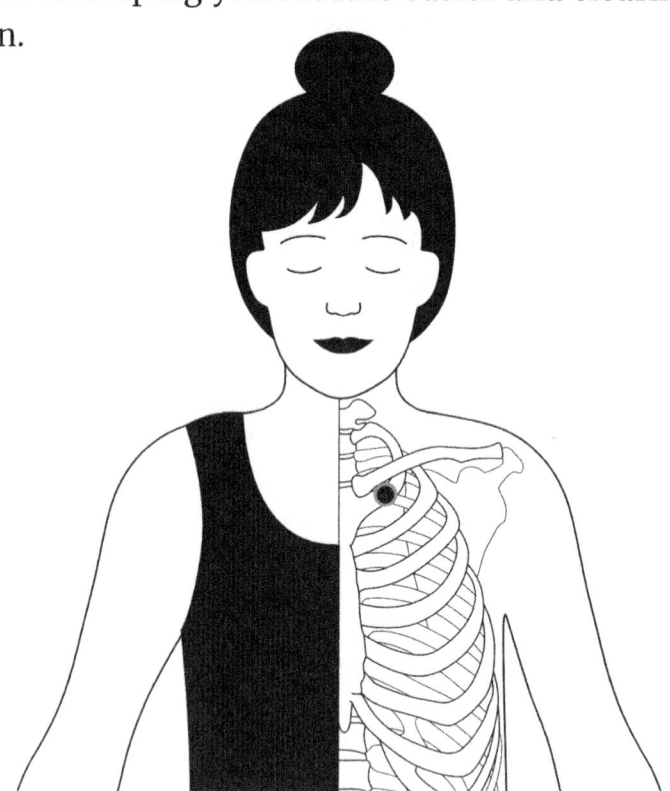

Location

Just below your collarbone, to the sides of your breastbone, you will feel hollows. Those hollows are the pressure points. This is a sensitive area, so you might feel more pain when applying pressure here than with the previous pressure points.

How To Stimulate The Acupoint

You can use one or both hands to activate acupoint KI 27. If you opt for 1 hand, you will use the tips of your thumb and middle finger. When using both hands, apply pressure with both middle fingers. As mentioned above, this is a sensitive area, so be gentle and use the fleshy parts of your fingertips instead of the ends.

Apply pressure and hold it for 30 seconds to 1 minute. Take 2 deep breaths and repeat the sequence 3 to 4 times. Make sure your shoulders and your body is relaxed the whole time.

Self-Reflection

After stimulating this acupoint, reflect on how you feel.

Date:_____

_____
_____
_____
_____
_____

Third Eye Acupoint (Governing Vessel 24.5)

The Third Eye Acupoint lies on the Governing Vessel channel and can also be referred to as GV 24.5. It is an effective point to stimulate if you want to relieve headaches and experience less stress. Some practitioners say that activating this point also helps alleviate eye strain and blocked sinuses.

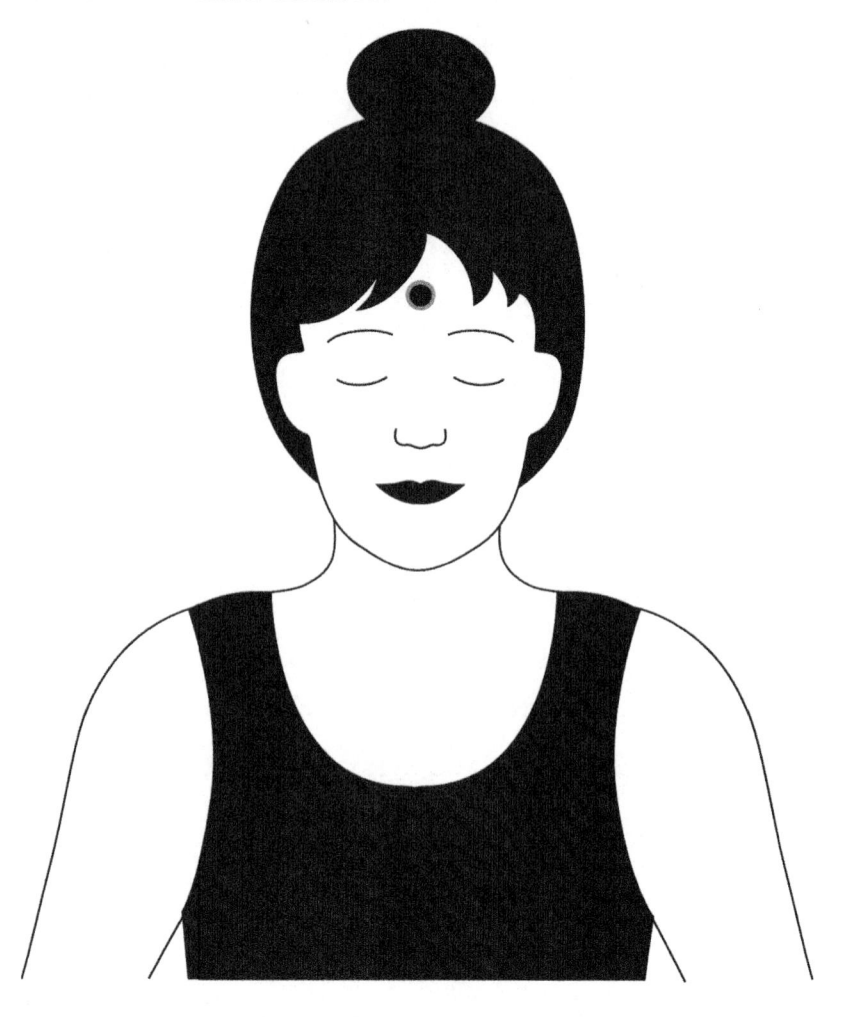

Location

You can find your Third Eye acupoint one finger width above the mid-point between your eyebrows.

How To Stimulate The Acupoint

Apply firm pressure to the acupoint for 2 to 3 minutes, or apply pressure while gently massaging the acupoint in a circular motion for 2 to 3 minutes.

> ## Self-Reflection
>
> After stimulating this acupoint, reflect on how you feel.
>
> Date:_____
>
> _____
> _____
> _____
> _____
> _____
> _____
> _____
> _____
> _____
> _____

Leg Three Mile Acupoint (Stomach 36)

This is one of the more popular and widely-used acupressure points. It lies on the Stomach energy channel and is also called ST 36. When stimulating this acupoint regularly, it can reduce fatigue and depression. It can also relieve pain anywhere in your body. The name 'Leg Three Mile' is a direct translation from its Chinese name, 'Zu San Li in Pinyin'. According to Chinese tradition, stimulating this acupoint is so powerful that it will let you walk 3 more miles when you're completely exhausted. It is also excellent in helping your body fight digestive issues like irritable bowel syndrome, nausea and vomiting, and diarrhoea.

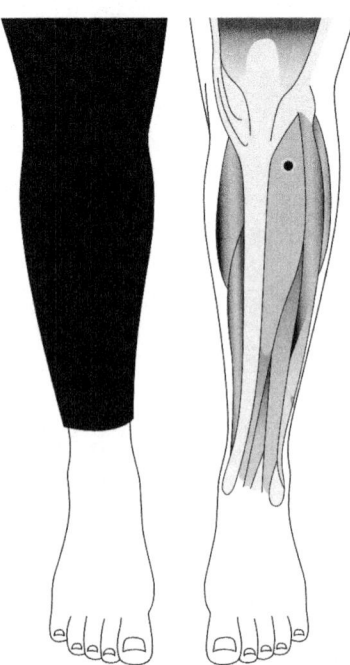

Location

The ST 36 point can be found on the front of both your lower legs. Place your palm over the kneecap, fingers extended down the lower leg. Your pinkie finger should be resting around the outside of your shin bone. Using your other hand, feel for the depression just below the end of your pinkie finger to the side of your shin bone. The depression is the acupoint.

How To Stimulate The Acupoint

Start pressing on the point gently and gradually increase the pressure. As you increase the pressure, move your finger slowly, too. Keep up the session for 2 to 3 minutes.

Self-Reflection

After stimulating this acupoint, reflect on how you feel.

Date:_____

_____

_____

_____

_____

_____

One Hundred Meeting Point Acupoint

This acupoint also lies on the Governing Vessel channel and is well known by its shorthand name, GV 20. Stimulating this point in your body brings about a sense of calm, relaxation, and enhanced creativity. It is also useful for sharpening your concentration.

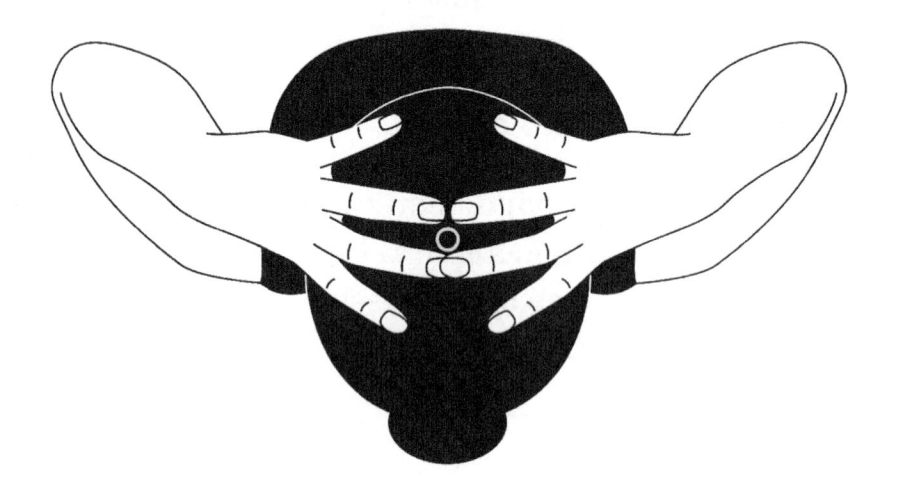

Location

Place the palm of your hands over your ears with the middle finger pointing upwards. Slide your middle fingers upwards till they touch in the midline at the highest point of the skull. There may be an indentation here, this is the acupoint.

How To Stimulate The Acupoint

As you engage in this acupressure session, concentrate on your breathing and make sure you are inhaling and exhaling deeply. Place a middle finger on the acupoint and press down until you feel an ache. Note that this should not be an ache that causes discomfort. While pressing down, close your eyes and continue to focus on your breathing. Keep up with the session for 2 to 3 minutes.

Self-Reflection

After stimulating this acupoint, reflect on how you feel.

Date:_____

_____
_____
_____

Shoulder well Acupoint (Gallbladder 21)

Also known as Gallbladder 21 or GB 21, this acupoint can relieve nervous tension, neck stiffness and headaches. It clears the head and calms the mind.

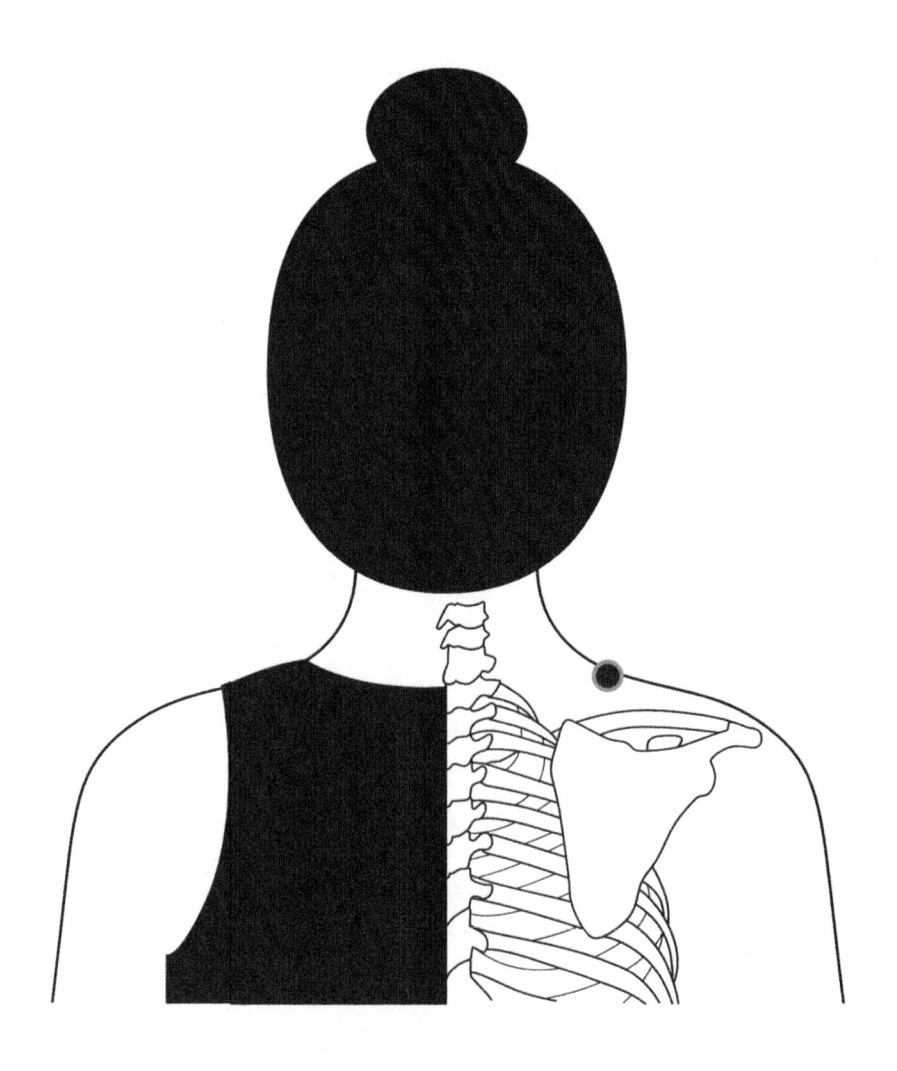

Location

You'll find GB 21 midway between the base of your neck and your outer shoulder, at the highest point on the shoulder muscle which is called the Trapezius.

How To Stimulate The Acupoint

Curve your hand over the opposite shoulder. Once you feel that tense muscle as described above, make sure your arm and shoulders are relaxed and then press down on that spot with firm pressure for 2 to 3 minutes. Take deep breaths while practising the technique. Shoulder muscles can be sensitive, so if you can't press it for 3 minutes at a time, try pressing it for 30 seconds to 1 minute, release it for a few seconds, and press again. Repeat the sequence 2 to 3 times.

Self-Reflection

After stimulating this acupoint, reflect on how you feel.

Date:_____
_____
_____
_____
_____
_____

Inner Gate Acupoint (Pericardium 6)

Inner Gate lies on the Pericardium channel and can also be referred to as P 6. It is an excellent point to stimulate when feeling nauseous and anxious. Furthermore, it is effective in alleviating bloating, tummy aches, and menstrual discomfort and pain. Some people who regularly stimulate this acupoint also report feeling more emotionally stable and calm in challenging situations.

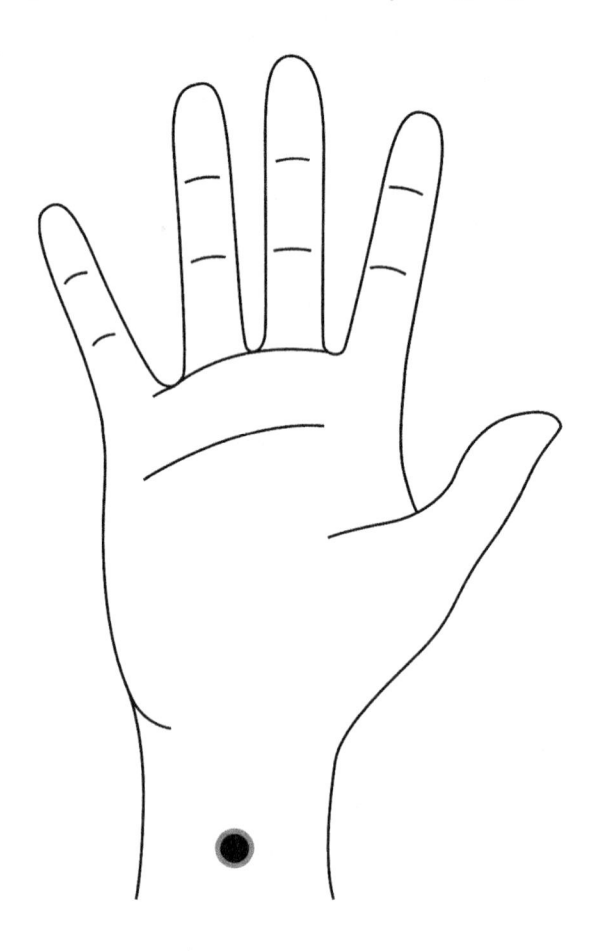

Location

Turn your hand palm to the sky. Place the 3 long fingers against the crease of your wrist, the outside of the index finger marks the distance from the wrist crease. The acupoint lies between the two tendons in the middle of the wrist.

How To Stimulate The Acupoint

Use your thumb to gently massage the acupoint for 30 seconds to 1 minute and take a 5-second break. Repeat this sequence 2 to 3 times.

Self-Reflection

After stimulating this acupoint, reflect on how you feel.

Date:_____

_____
_____
_____
_____
_____
_____
_____

Shining Sea Acupoint (Kidney 6)

Shenmai acupoint (Bl 62) that we discussed earlier basically sits at the opposite side of the Shining Sea acupoint (also called KI 6). Together, they work wonders to help you obtain peaceful and meaningful sleep. While Bl 62 lies on the Bladder channel, KI 6 lies on the Kidney channel. Stimulating this acupoint nourishes your kidneys, calms your mind, and benefits your eyes, throat, and uterus.

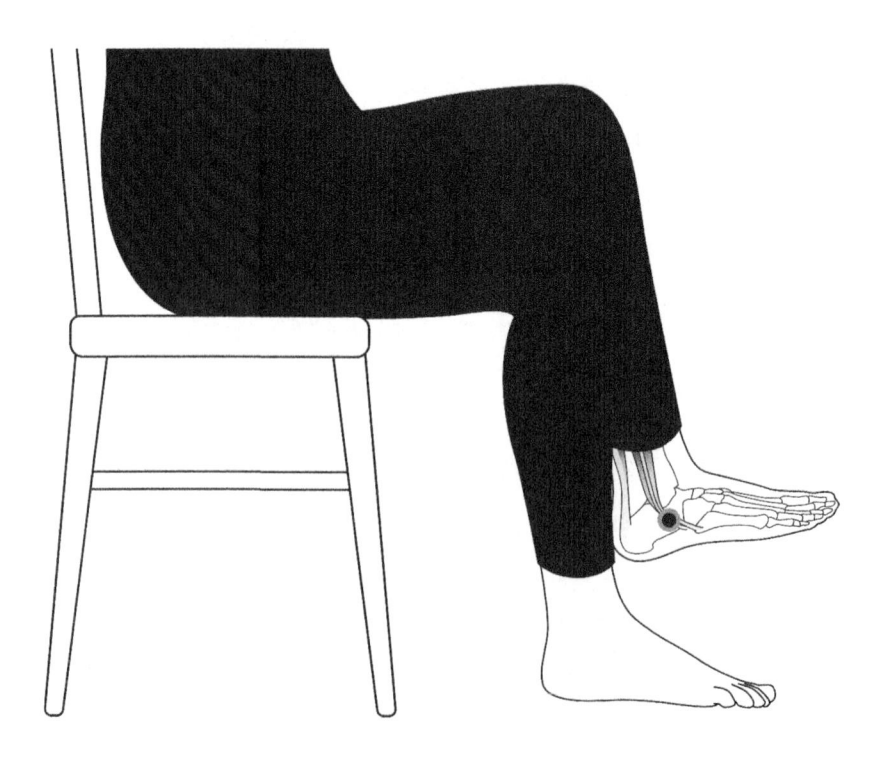

Location

You can find this acupoint in the hollow just beneath your inner ankle bone.

How To Stimulate The Acupoint

Use your thumbs to apply firm pressure on the acupoint for 2 to 3 minutes just before you go to sleep or if you need to calm your nerves in a stressful situation.

Self-Reflection

After stimulating this acupoint, reflect on how you feel.

Date:_____
_____
_____
_____
_____
_____
_____
_____
_____
_____

Central Mansion Acupoint (Lung 1)

The fact that this acupoint lies on the Lung energy channel is apt, as letting go of pent-up feelings and negativity is as liberating as releasing a deep breath you have been holding in. It is also called LU 1. The Letting Go acupoint can help you manage feelings of frustration, distress, and anxiety. It can also alleviate chest pain, difficulty breathing, coughing, and wheezing.

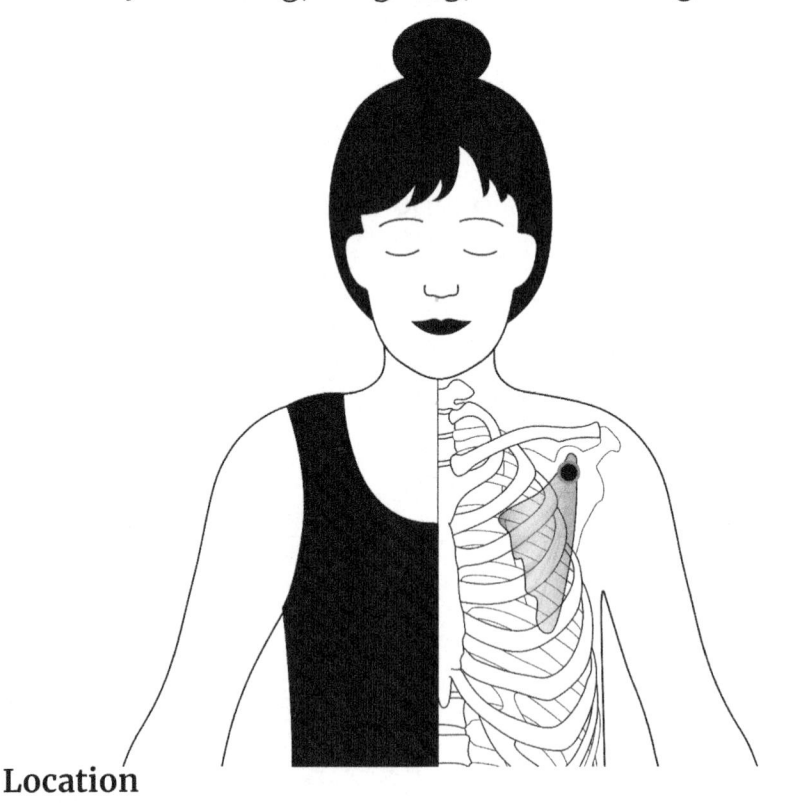

Location

You can find LU 1 in between your first and second ribs toward the outer chest. Extend 4 fingers (not including your thumb) and place them so your index finger rests against the bottom edge of your clavicle (or collar bone).

The acupoint lies in the area where your pinkie finger rests.

Feel around until you find the most tender point in a hollow.

How To Stimulate The Acupoint

You can activate LU 1 with firm pressure for 2 to 3 minutes or by tapping the acupoint for the same amount of time. However, when doing this the first few times, we would recommend you stick to just applying pressure. Once you know exactly where the acupoint lies, you can experiment with the tapping technique.

Self-Reflection

After stimulating this acupoint, reflect on how you feel.

Date: _____

_____
_____
_____
_____
_____
_____
_____

Middle Of Person Acupoint (Governing Vessel 26)

The Middle of Person acupoint, or GV 26, lies on the Governing Vessel channel. This acupoint is especially potent in heightening your alertness. If you find yourself feeling drowsy or 'out of it' in the middle of the day or when you really ought to be concentrating, this is the perfect remedy. In addition to alertness, it can also relieve dizziness. There have been cases where people were revived from fainting after receiving acupressure on the Middle of Person Acupoint. It can also uplift your spirit and clear brain fog.

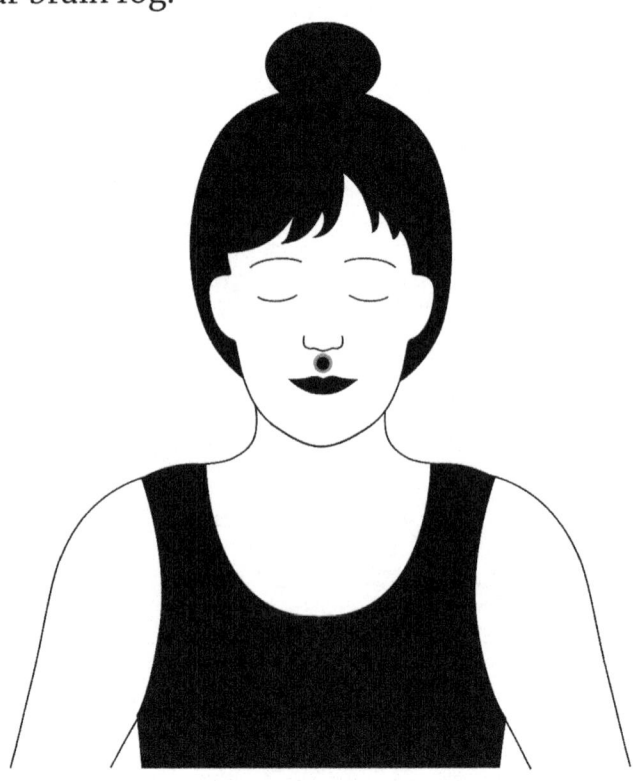

Location

GV 26 sits at the base of the nose in the groove joining the base of the nose to the upper lip.

How To Stimulate The Acupoint

Press down firmly just below the base of your nose and then slightly shift the pressure upward. Hold the pressure for around 2 minutes.

Self-Reflection

After stimulating this acupoint, reflect on how you feel.

Date:_____

_____
_____
_____
_____
_____
_____
_____
_____
_____

Spirit Gate Acupoint (Heart 7)

Also called H 7, the Spirit Gate acupoint lies on the Heart energy channel. This acupoint has the power to ground your emotions and bring back the feeling of being balanced and in control. It helps your body fight against anxiety, depression, and insomnia. You can also lower your heart rate in situations that cause you a lot of stress or irritation.

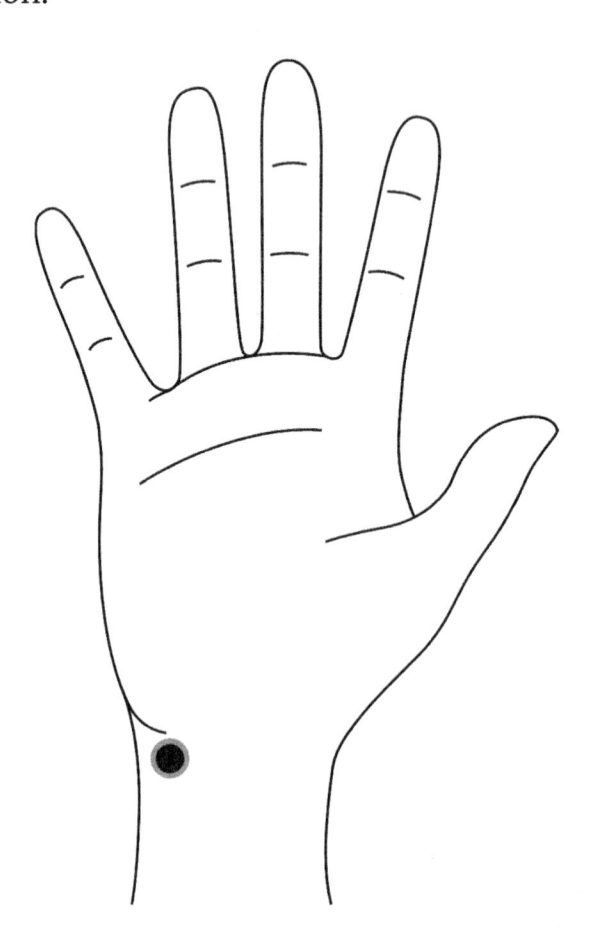

Location

H 7 lies on your outer wrist. Draw an imaginary line from the inside of your pinky to the crease of your wrist. There is a slight depression, which is the spot of this acupoint.

How To Stimulate The Acupoint

Apply firm pressure to the acupoint for 2 to 3 minutes, or gently massage it in a circular motion for 2 to 3 minutes.

Self-Reflection

After stimulating this acupoint, reflect on how you feel.

Date:_____
_____
_____
_____
_____
_____
_____
_____
_____
_____

Kidney Shu Acupoint (Bladder 23)

Sea of Vitality, or Bl 23, is yet another point on the Bladder energy channel. Stimulate this point to combat fatigue and irritability. You can also use it to reduce lower back pain and strengthen your core.

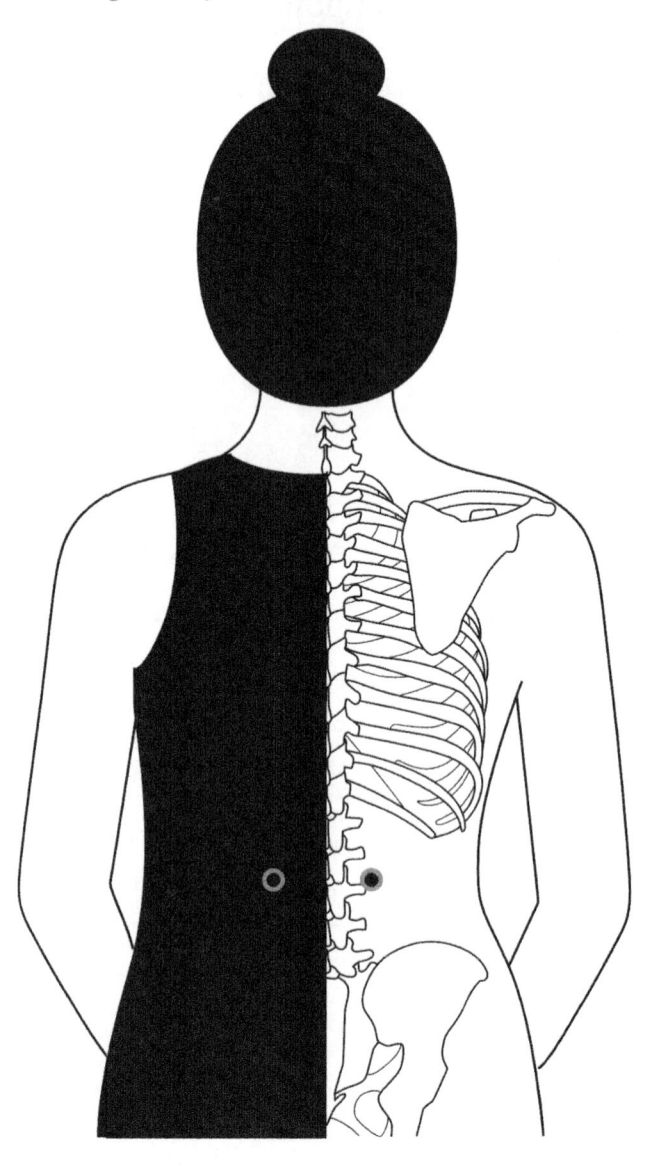

Location

B 23 sits just about waist-high on your lower back. To find it, place your hands around your waist, index finger against the edge of your lower ribs. Now extend your thumbs to your back. The acupoint sits on both sides of the spine, about an inch away from its edges to either side.

How To Stimulate The Acupoint

Whenever you are working on or near your spine, be careful not to apply too much pressure. Use your thumbs to massage both sides of the B 23 acupoint firmly but gently for 2 to 3 minutes.

Self-Reflection

After stimulating this acupoint, reflect on how you feel.

Date:_____

_____

_____

_____

_____

_____

_____

Rest Bite Takeaway

I have shared quite a handful of acupressure techniques above. However, you need not feel pressured to learn all of them at once.

Take 10 to 15 minutes to identify the two most pressing issues you are currently facing in terms of your emotional and physical health. Write them down and read through the above techniques again. This time, pick 2 or 3 of the techniques that will make the most difference in your life right now. Once you have your techniques, start implementing them at least once a day at a time that best suits your situation.

Acupressure Sequences For Everyday Mum Challenges

Treat each of the following sequences as 15-minute Rest Bites you can incorporate into your life. As suggested above, identify what you need most at the moment and start using those techniques first. As you get more comfortable with self-acupressure, you can implement more techniques.

Since I have already explained each acupressure point, I will not repeat the information here. Instead, I'll list which sequence of points works best for the given issue. If you need to refresh your memory on how to stimulate each point, head back to the previous section for a quick read.

You will get the most out of these sequences if you spend 3 to 5 minutes on each acupoint, alternating between applying fixed pressure and firm massaging motions. For each of the sequences, find a space where you can sit comfortably. Keep your shoulders relaxed the entire time, make sure your spine is straight, and take deep, calm breaths as you do the sequences.

Calming Self-Acupressure

- Upper Sea of Qi (CV 17)
- Spirit Gate (H 7)
- Third Eye (GV 24.5)

Energy Boosting Self-Acupressure

- Shenmai (Bl 62)
- Three-mile point (ST 36)
- Middle of Person (GV 26)

Sleep Support Self-Acupressure

- Shining sea (KI 6)

- Upper Sea of Qi(CV 17)
- Shenmai (Bl 62)

Stress Relief Self-Acupressure

- Central mansion (LU 1)
- Spirit Gate (H 7)
- Inner Gate (P 6)

Memory And Focus Self-Acupressure

- One Hundred Meeting Point (GV 20)
- Kidny Shu (B 23)
- Spirit Gate (H 7)

Calming Feelings Of Irritability And Frustration Self-Acupressure

- Central mansion (LU 1)
- Middle of Person (GV 26)
- Shu mansion(K 27)

Final Thoughts On Self-Acupressure

The truth is that you have nothing to lose by trying these techniques. They require almost no effort and will not waste the little time you have. In the end, you're the mama-bear, and you're the one who must decide what's best for you and your family.

That said, you might just discover that there is literal magic in self-acupressure that can help you navigate your days with just a little more ease. Try it— and if it doesn't work for you, you have many more tools in your self-care arsenal.

> When you recover or discover something that nourishes your soul and brings you joy, care enough about yourself to make room for it in your life.
>
> (Jean Shinoda Bole)

Use the space below to write down any thoughts or feelings you are experiencing right now. Be sure to add a date so you can see how much you've grown as a person when you come across this page in the future.

Chapter 7
Restorative Yoga For Rest

For those unfamiliar with yoga, it is easy to assume that 'Yoga is just stretching'. In reality, though, you get quite a few different types of Yoga.

Before exploring the type of Yoga I believe is best for mums, I'd like to give you a brief overview of what Yoga is, as there are so many theories and opinions on it these days.

What Is Yoga?

Yoga comes down to a practice of the body and mind. When practising Yoga, you use a combination of movements, meditation, and breathing techniques as a means of promoting your emotional, physical, and spiritual well-being.

A Brief History Of Yoga

Yoga is an ancient practice, dating back at least 5,000 years. The earliest documents and manuscripts describing Yoga come from India. Looking into Western history, it looks like it came to our culture during the 1890s via Indian monks. As with many other Eastern healing practices, Yoga became popular in the West during the 1970s when there was a surge of interest in alternative medicine and health practices.

Benefits Of Practising Yoga

There have been many scientific studies to understand the effects of Yoga on people's physical and mental health. It shows promise in various aspects of human health and, because of the widespread interest in Yoga, more and more studies are being conducted each year.

Let's look at how yoga can benefit you from a scientific point of view.

- Yoga increases flexibility (in fact, it is one of the top reasons people practise it).
- Yoga increases your body strength.
- Practising yoga regularly reduces inflammation in your body, thereby reducing your risk of developing

serious conditions like arthritis, heart disease, and digestive diseases.

- It is effective in relieving stress
- It can help to improve your mental health
- There is a link between practising Yoga and improved immunity.
- Yoga has shown to improve sleep in people suffering from anxiety and mild insomnia.
- The poses involved in Yoga can strengthen your bones (women are more susceptible to osteoporosis, so this is a big one).
- Yoga promotes better posture.
- Yoga can help prevent and manage burnout.

The Best Type Of Yoga For Mums

One branch of yoga, Hatha yoga, is concerned with improving your physical and mental wellness. It is also the branch most people in the West practise. Within this branch is a type of Yoga that, I believe greatly benefits new mums. The name says it all: Restorative yoga.

When practising restorative yoga, the focus is not so much on physical strengthening. It is all about letting go by releasing pent-up muscle tension and stimulating your organs slightly. You achieve this through long-held poses that are not strenuous but supportive and comfortable for your body.

Restorative Yoga is all about re-learning how to relax and be still. It's an effective way to develop self-soothing skills, enhance your capacity to heal physically and emotionally, and bring back balance to your nervous system so you can manage the stresses of life better.

Your autonomic nervous system (functions you do not need to control, like your heartbeat or the production of hormones) has 2 branches, called the parasympathetic nervous system and the sympathetic nervous system. Both systems affect the same body functions, including your heart rate, awareness, muscle tension, and reaction time. However, the ways in which they affect these functions differ like night and day. The parasympathetic nervous system is responsible for inducing a state of calm in your body and allows your body to rest and repair itself. The sympathetic nervous system, on the other hand, is responsible for the infamous 'fight or flight' mode that gears your body to react to perceived threats. Where the parasympathetic nervous system slows down your heart rate and eases your mind, the sympathetic nervous system increases your heart rate and makes you alert so you can respond to stress at a moment's notice.

No one has control over the autonomic nervous system—it just responds to whatever is happening in our direct environments. And, as you know, stress in the right doses is important, because it's that stress that motivates you to take appropriate action. While you cannot control your nervous system, you can teach yourself to analyse perceived threats better, thereby allowing your body to respond better in stressful situations and to switch between the sympathetic and parasympathetic modes with more ease.

For example, if you have a disagreement with your partner and your autonomic nervous system is not in balance, you may end up having a terrible day altogether because of your body's inability to switch from the sympathetic mode (fight or flight) to the parasympathetic mode (calm) once the disagreement is over.

This is where restorative yoga works wonders. Practising this type of yoga will help you be more in touch with your parasympathetic nervous system and give your body the means to move between the parasympathetic and sympathetic states more easily. By re-learning the art of relaxation through restorative yoga, you can help your body produce less stress hormones, reduce sleeplessness, improve your immunity, and reduce muscle tensions that cause headaches and other body aches and pains.

Is Restorative Yoga Really For You?

If you can answer 'yes' to any one of the following questions, restorative Yoga can benefit you tremendously.

- Do you have a hard time falling asleep at night?

- Do you feel tired when you wake up in the morning?

- Has your road rage been a little out of control lately?

- Are you not able to turn off your worried brain no matter what you do?

- Do you need a little less chaos in your life?

- Can you not stop 'multitasking' even when you shouldn't be doing it?

Rest Bite Takeaway

If you're feeling a bit overwhelmed with all the self-care techniques you have learned so far, take a deep breath and a step back.

Remember that you need not use all the techniques all the time. They're tools to help you fight exhaustion and get through your days and should not be a source of extra concern. If you haven't started using a technique by now, take time to identify the greatest source of frustration in your life at the moment. Chances are, there is a technique in this book that can bring relief. For now, focus on practising that technique only.

Best Restorative Poses With Minimal Props

Restorative yoga employs many props to increase your level of comfort while practising it. These props include bolsters, blankets, and pillows among other tools. As wonderful as the props are in their contribution to making you feel nourished and supporting a restful pose, they're not the most practical thing for new mums. Using everything restorative yoga suggests takes up space, time, and resources you may not have. So, I chose the poses that require the least amount of props (or no props at all) that will be most effective yet easy to do.

Child's Pose (Balasana)

In yoga, the child's pose is the ultimate resting posture. It is the perfect start for those who have never practised yoga before, as it puts minimal strain on your muscles. Despite its gentleness, it is very effective.

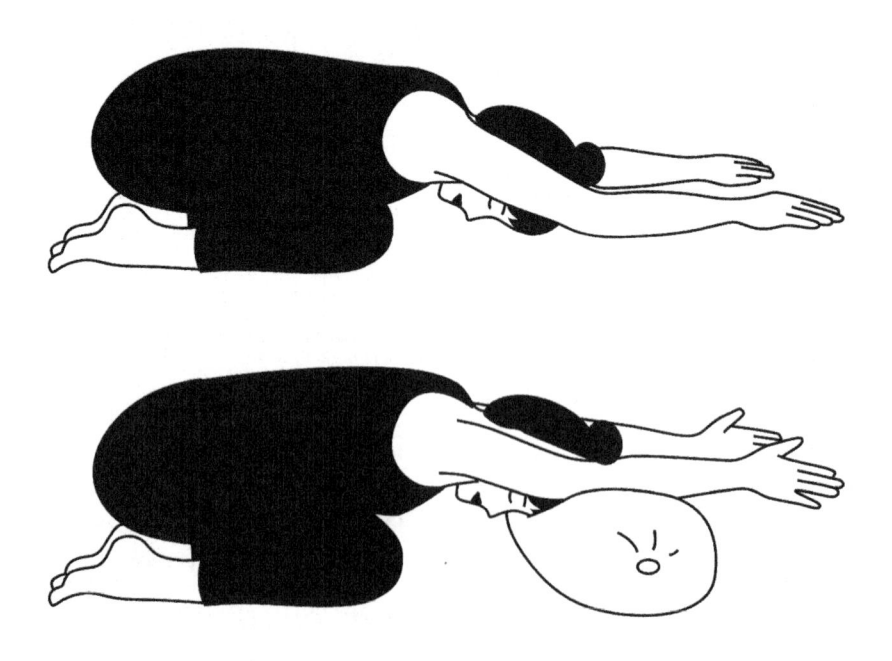

Self-Reflection

Before doing the Child's Pose, reflect on how you feel physically and emotionally.

Date:_____

_____
_____
_____
_____
_____
_____
_____
_____
_____
_____
_____
_____
_____
_____
_____
_____
_____

How To Do The Child's Pose

The child's pose does not require props and can be done in as much or as little time as you need. So, whenever you need an instant rest break, this can be your go-to self-care ritual.

Step 1

Sit on your heels and spread your knees apart slightly, keeping your big toes touching. Your knees should be apart far enough for your torso to fit in between them.

Step 2

Take a deep breath. As you slowly exhale, start leaning forward until your forehead rests on the floor, and your torso is between your knees. You can extend your arms overhead and let your palms rest on the floor, or you can rest your arms alongside your body with your palms facing upward as they rest on the floor.

Step 3

Relax your tailbone toward your heels. If your hips feel uncomfortably tight, take your knees further apart from each other. You may feel like your knees need extra support, in which case you can place a folded blanket underneath you for the pose.

Step 4

While holding the pose, bring all your thoughts inward until you're focused on your breathing only. Feel the natural flow of your body's inhaling and exhaling. Try to extend your exhaling as far as you can. Take note of tension in your body and try to breathe into those tight spaces as much as possible.

Variations Of The Child's Pose

Side Stretch Child's Pose

With your arms extended overhead, you can do lovely and surprisingly satisfying side stretches during this pose. Before you do side stretches, always start with the regular child's pose to relax your body.

Let your hands 'walk' to the one side of your body. For a deep stretch, you can try to bring the opposite hand over the other, (for example, if you're stretching to the left, bring your right hand over your left hand). Continue taking deep breaths as you stretch. Be mindful of the hip opposite the direction you are stretching in; if it lifts, try to guide it back against the floor. When you're ready, repeat the stretch on the other side.

Supported Child's Pose

Before you enter the child's pose, place a bolster vertically in front of you. As you move into position, the bolster will offer support between your knees and give your torso a comfortable resting platform. Let your head rest against the bolster to one side. Take at least ten deep breaths before you turn your head to the other side and do the same.

Another version of the supported child's pose is to place the bolster horizontally in front of you. After entering the pose, fold your arms on the bolster to allow complete relaxation of your neck, jaw, and shoulders.

Child's Pose Benefits

Physical Benefits

The child's pose gives your hips, back, thighs, and ankles a gentle stretch. It is especially effective in elongating your lower back and keeping your hip muscles flexible. Because of modern life (we sit way more than our ancestors), lower backs and hips are suffering the world over. It is important to take time during the day to nurture those critical muscles to ensure less pain as you grow older.

With regular practise, you can promote healthy digestion and strengthen your knees. The pose also stimulates circulation to your spine, organs, and brain.

Emotional And Mental Benefits

The moment you enter this position, your brain receives signals that you are safe and it knows that it is OK to switch into rest mode. In this pose, your forehead will rest on the floor, activating your Third Eye acupoint, thereby inducing a state of calm even further. The child's pose is, in essence, a restorative and rejuvenating activity for both your mind and body.

When To Avoid The Child's Pose:

- If you have diarrhoea;
- during pregnancy;
- if you have a serious knee injury.

Self-Reflection

After doing the Child's Pose, reflect on how you feel physically and emotionally.

Date:_____

_____
_____
_____
_____
_____
_____
_____
_____

Legs Up The Wall Pose

This pose relaxes your mind and encourages your body to switch into the parasympathetic mode. It's the perfect remedy after a long day (or night—if your baby kept you up), or if you're just feeling tired, frustrated, or stressed.

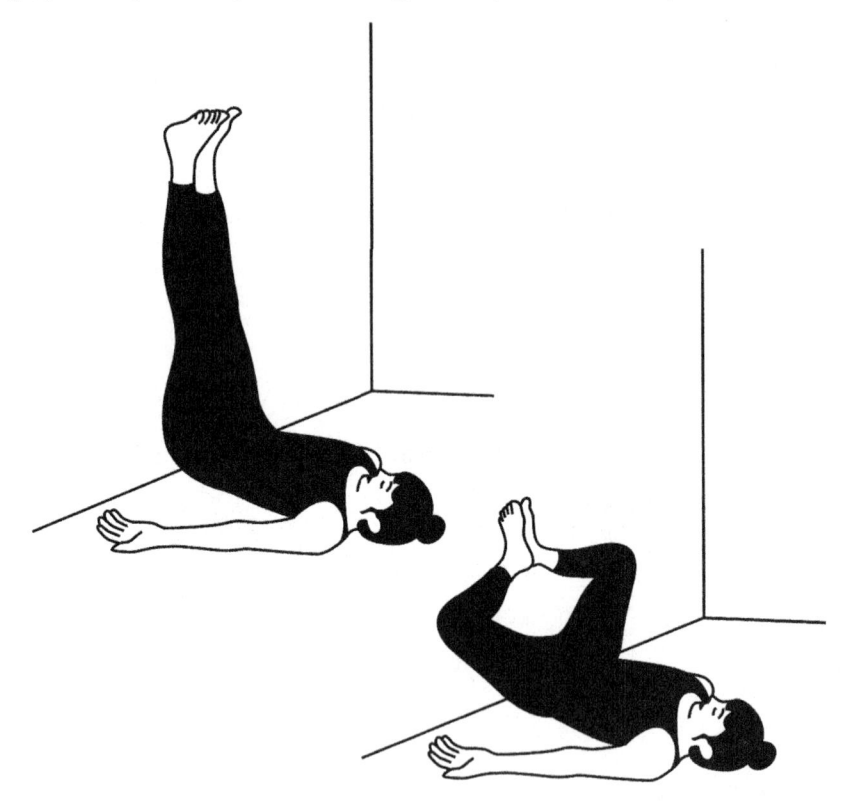

Self-Reflection

Before doing the Legs Up the Wall Pose, reflect on how you feel physically and emotionally.

Date:_____

_____
_____
_____
_____
_____
_____
_____
_____
_____
_____
_____
_____
_____
_____
_____
_____
_____
_____

How To Do The Legs Up The Wall Pose

You'll need a wall, a yoga mat, and a blanket for this pose. The yoga mat will increase your comfort, as you'll be holding the pose for at least 5minutes. However, if you do not have a yoga mat, you can use blankets as an alternative. As you move into position, make sure the blankets don't form creases that can cause discomfort.

Step 1

With your knees bent and ankles drawn inward, sit on the floor with your right or left side about 5 inches from the wall.

Step 2

Turn your body toward the wall and lie down. While entering this position, swing your legs upward so they rest against the wall. If you do not have a yoga mat you can lie on, place your blanket underneath your hip area before you lie down.

Step 3

Relax your pelvis, so your back does not arch. If you are flexible, you can scoot your hips until they're up against the wall, with your legs extended straight above your hips, but don't push yourself to do this if you're less flexible. It's all about feeling comfortable while practising this pose.

Step 4

Let your hands rest next to your body or on your stomach. Relax your neck and face and take deep breaths. Hold the pose for 5 to 10 minutes. When you're done, gently bend your knees and swing your legs to the side of the wall and let them rest on the floor. Lie for 30 seconds to a minute before you get up.

Good To Know

You may experience tingling in your legs or feet while doing the Legs up the Wall pose. If this happens to you, gently bend your knees and draw them toward your chest. Next, roll to one of your sides. You can end the exercise right there or have another go at the pose, depending on how relaxed you feel.

Variations Of The Legs Up The Wall Pose

Turn It Into A Breathing Exercise

You can enhance the relaxing experience by focusing on your breathing like you do with the Child's Pose. Find a formula that works for you; for example, inhale for a count of 4 and exhale for a count of 6. The longer you can exhale, the more your nervous system will relax.

Keep up the breathing exercise for as long as you feel comfortable with it, and then rest by maintaining the pose until you feel you're ready to continue with your day.

Butterfly Pose

Push your soles against each other, bend your knees, and draw them toward your hips (while keeping your legs against the wall).

The Butterfly alternative allows for a deeper stretch of your hips and thighs.

Do You Have Busy Hands?

If you are prone to fidgeting with your hands and don't know what to do with them while practising the Legs Up the Wall pose, consider stimulating acupoints on your wrists, like the Inner Gate or Spirit gate.

Legs Up The Wall Pose Benefits

Physical Benefits

Practising the Legs up the Wall pose reduces swelling in your legs, ankles, and feet and improves circulation, especially if you spend many consecutive hours seated or on your feet. If you suffer from foot and leg cramps, this pose will also bring relief. Here are some more scientifically-backed benefits:

- It's good for your thyroid function;
- it relieves headaches and migraines;
- it helps to regulate your blood pressure;

- you can manage varicose veins with this pose;

- it helps to manage lower back pain;

- the pose improves the flow of lymph fluid, thereby boosting your immunity.

Emotional And Mental Benefits

This is a calming pose that allows your body to release pent-up tension. If you experience a lot of stress, anxiety, or even depression, practising this pose on a regular basis can help you manage it better. It can also help to regulate and improve your sleeping habits.

When To Avoid The Legs Up The Wall Pose

- If you have glaucoma, as the pose can increase the fluid pressure in your eyes.

- If you struggle with excessive fluid retention in your body. If you have high blood pressure that is not being managed properly.

- If you have respiratory, spinal, or heart issues, or a serious eye condition, it's best to talk with your doctor before doing this pose.

- Avoid this pose while menstruating.

- If you are past 3 months of pregnancy. (Also, avoid this pose for the first 3 months after your pregnancy).

- Wait for at least 2 hours after a meal before you do the Legs Up the Wall pose.

Self-Reflection

After doing the Legs Up the Wall Pose, reflect on how you feel physically and emotionally.

Date:_____

_____
_____
_____
_____
_____
_____
_____
_____
_____
_____
_____
_____
_____

Seated Forward Bend

If you are having a particularly challenging day and feel very anxious, the Seated Forward bend has the potential to bring immediate relief. Restorative yoga (and Yoga in general) is as much a mindfulness technique as it is physical. Practising it the right way requires all your attention, which allows you to redirect your thoughts from reliving bad experiences and thinking of little irritations to enjoying an intimate moment with yourself.

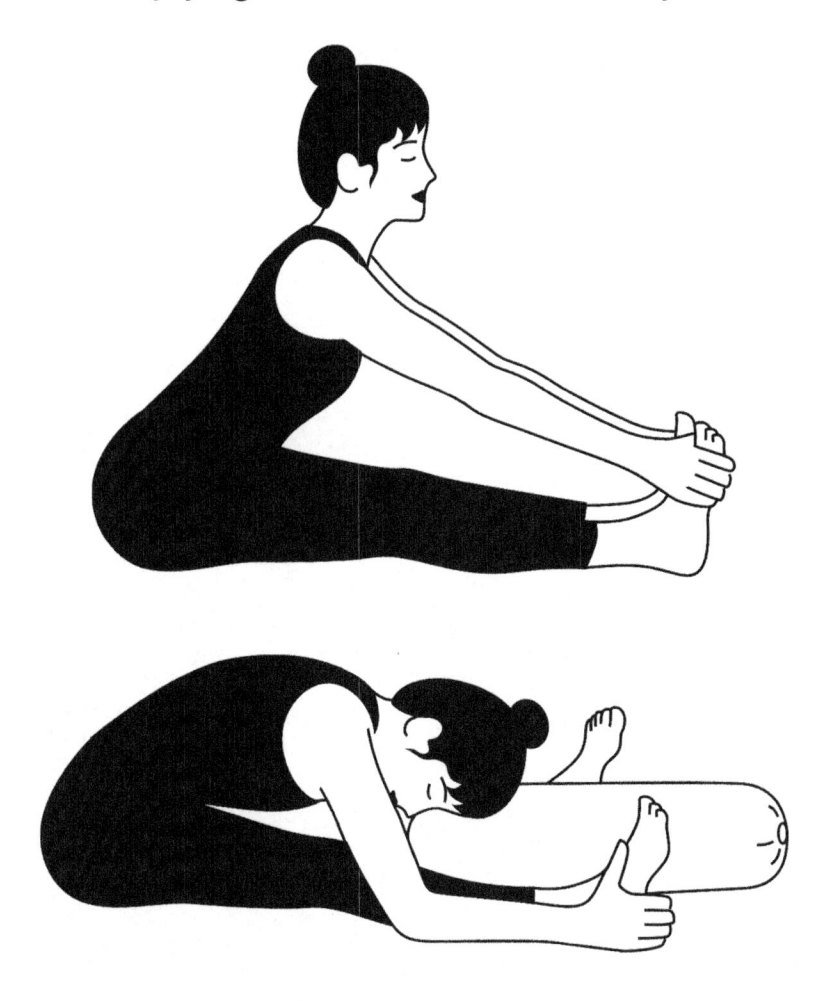

Self-Reflection

Before doing the Seated Forward Bend, reflect on how you feel physically and emotionally.

Date:

How To Do The Seated Forward Bend

All you need to benefit from this pose is 30 seconds to 2 minutes. You can use this technique whenever you need to reconnect with yourself and find a place of calm. If you can, try this technique at least 3 times a day.

Step 1

Go to one of your favourite spots in the house and find a place to sit on the floor. Fold a blanket and place it underneath you, so your hips are raised slightly.

Step 2

Push your legs out in front of you so they extend all the way and make sure your back remains straight.

Step 3

Raise your arms into the air and inhale, taking in as much breath as possible. As you exhale, let your torso move forward slightly as if to fold onto your lower body, but be sure to keep your back straight so it does not round as you move.

Step 4

Bend your knees ever so slightly, flex your toes, and lift your kneecaps a little. Doing this protects your knees while still allowing an effective stretch for your hamstrings.

With each inhalation, extend your spine a little more to lean into the pose further. The trick is to keep your spine straight the entire time.

Do not try to fold over all the way if your muscles are not flexible enough to achieve it. Instead, go as far as your body allows and take your time.

Step 5

When your body has gone as far as it can, let your arms rest next to your legs. If your palms face toward the floor, you will activate more grounding, and if they face upward, you will activate more receptivity. While grounding and receptivity are both powerful, I am especially appreciative of the latter, as it allows you to feel what is true for you at the moment. Being in a receptive state releases patterns of tension and allows you to feel all you need without judgement.

Variations Of The Seated Forward Bend

Seated Head To Knee Pose

Start the pose as explained in steps 1 and 2 of the Seated Forward Bend. Keeping your spine straight, bend one leg until the bent leg's sole rests against the inside of the other upper leg. Take a deep breath and start leaning your torso forward, but be sure to keep your spine straight. Every time you exhale, extend your spine a little more. Your goal is to bring your head closer to your straight leg's knee. If you can manage to reach your foot, hold onto it during the pose; otherwise, let your arms relax alongside your extended leg. Lengthen your spine as much as your body allows and then hold the pose for as long as you can.

Seated Forward Bend Benefits

Physical Benefits

This pose stretches your spine, shoulders, hamstrings, and calves. It is one of the best stretches to strengthen your lower back and keep those critical muscles flexible. It also stimulates and nourishes your digestive system, together with your kidneys, liver, ovaries, and uterus.

Emotional And Mental Benefits

Like the Child's Pose, the Seated Forward Bend immediately signals to your brain that it's safe to unwind. This induces a state of calm that helps you deal with anxiety and mild depression.

When To Avoid The Seated Forward Bend

- If you have a back injury, no matter how mild, avoid this pose. (You can, however, practise it under professional supervision if your doctor gives you the go-ahead.)
- Don't practise this pose if your pregnancy term is past 2 months.

- If you are menstruating, don't bend over too far. If you have diarrhoea, wait until it's over.

Yoga is a light, which once lit will never dim. The better your practise, the brighter your flame.

(B. K. S. Iyengar)

Self-Reflection

After doing the Seated Forward Bend, reflect on how you feel physically and emotionally.

Date:_____
_____
_____
_____
_____
_____
_____
_____
_____
_____

Easy Pose With Forward Fold

This is another calming and soothing pose for an exhausted and overactive mind. You can practise it on its own or as part of a sequence that includes the other calming poses you have already learned.

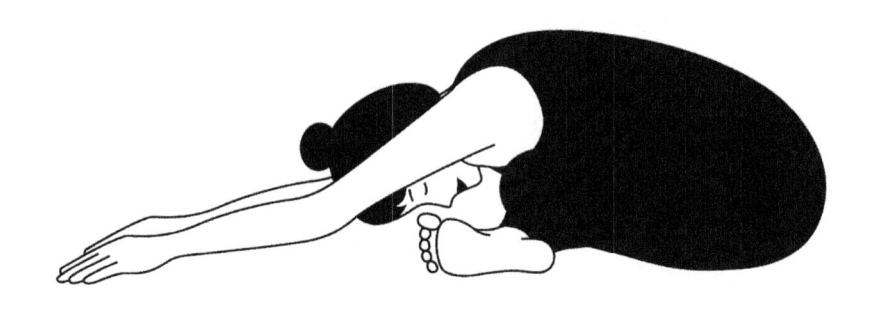

Rest Bite Takeaway

Remember that investing time, even a few minutes a day, in yourself is totally worth it and that you deserve it. You cannot give your partner and child the best of you if you can't even give it to yourself.

Self-Reflection

Before doing the Easy Pose with Forward Fold, reflect on how you feel physically and emotionally.

Date:_ _

_ _

_ _

_ _

_ _

_ _

_ _

_ _

_ _

_ _

_ _

_ _

_ _

_ _

_ _

How To Do The Easy Pose With Forward Fold

You'll find that the best time of day to practise this pose is in the morning or evening (you can even do it twice a day if you prefer).

Step 1

You'll start off by sitting on the ground. How much support your hips will need depends on how tight your hips are. The tighter they are, the more support I recommend, as it will make you much more comfortable. You can use folded blankets or a cushion as support props. Having the support will reduce the strain on your knees and help you properly align your spine during the pose.

Step 2

Cross your legs in front of you, with each foot resting more or less underneath its opposite knee. Shift your weight until your sitting bones are balanced evenly while making sure your spine, neck and head line up with each other. Take a deep breath and relax your thighs and feet as you exhale.

Step 3

Take another deep breath and lengthen your spine as you go. When you exhale, let your torso bow forward with your arms extended in front of you. Let your head rest on the floor and continue to take slow, deep breaths. You can fold your arms over each other to create some elevation and let them rest in front of your head.

If you find it difficult to bend all the way down, place a support prop like a yoga block, a pillow, or a chair in front of you for support.

Throughout the pose, be mindful that you do not round your back too much or hunch your shoulders. You want your spine to be extended and as straight as possible the entire time. Hold the pose for 3 to 5 minutes, and then switch your legs for another stretch of the same length.

Easy Pose With Forward Fold Benefits

Physical Benefits

Practising this pose will keep your hips mobile, strengthen your back, decompress your spine, open your chest, and relieve neck strain.

Emotional And Mental Benefits

You will feel more balanced, calm, and in control with the help of this self-care technique. It's also an effective way to fight stress-induced fatigue.

When To Avoid The Easy Pose With Forward Fold

- If you are suffering from any knee injuries.
- If you are pregnant.

- If your hips are very stiff, be cautious with this pose. Have enough support available to raise your hips, and don't force your body further than it feels comfortable to go.

Self-Reflection

After doing the Easy Pose with Forward Fold, reflect on how you feel physically and emotionally.

Date: _____
_____
_____
_____
_____
_____
_____
_____
_____
_____
_____
_____
_____
_____
_____

Laying Down Twist Pose

Also known as the supine spinal twist, it is the perfect pose to relax your whole body and bring everything into harmony after completing your other yoga poses.

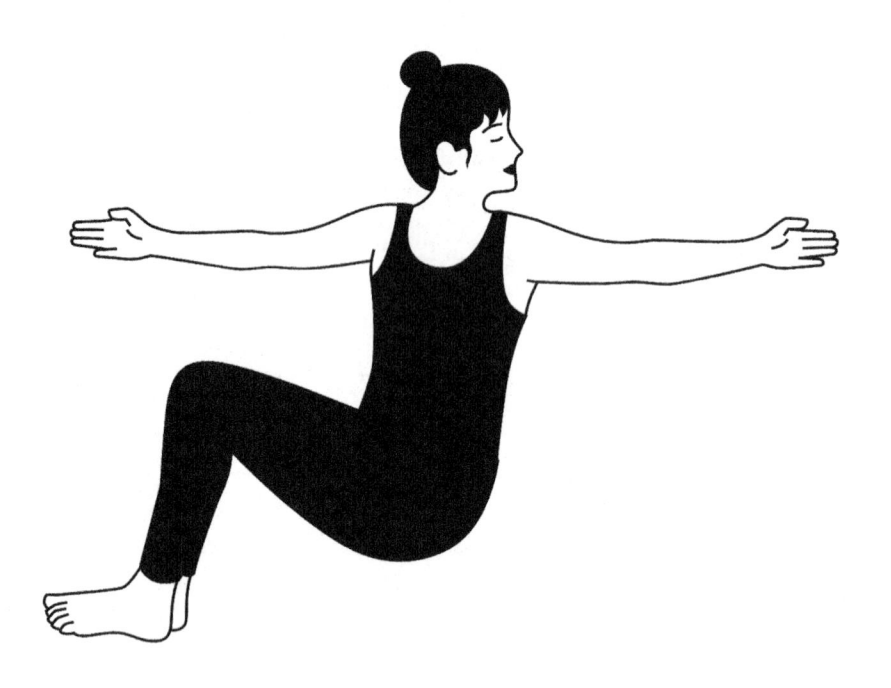

Self-Reflection

Before doing the Laying Down Twist Pose, reflect on how you feel physically and emotionally.

Date:_____

_____
_____
_____
_____
_____
_____
_____
_____
_____
_____
_____
_____
_____
_____
_____
_____
_____

How To Do The Laying Down Twist Pose

Step 1

Find a spot where you can lie down comfortably on your back. If you do not have a yoga mat to lie on, use a couple of blankets. Take a deep breath and relax the body with your next exhalation. Be especially mindful that your shoulders are flat on the ground and that you don't arch your back.

Step 2

Bend your knees and bring them up to your chest, let the weight of your knees be supported by your hands. Begin to rock from side to side, then continue by gentle movements backwards and forwards to give your back a soothing massage. After about 2-3 minutes of exploring these movements, come to stillness.

Step 3

Let your arms rest in a t-position, palms facing downward. On your next exhalation, bring your bent knees to the right side.

Step 4

Relax your whole body and continue to take slow, deep breaths while resting in this position. As you breathe, be mindful of the tight areas in your lower back and between your shoulders. With each inhalation, guide your breath into those spaces, and with each exhalation, feel the softening in your body.

Stay in the pose for 3 to 5 minutes, then switch sides and bring your knees the other way.

Good to Know

If your body is tense because of life's daily stresses, you might notice your shoulders lifting as you twist your spine. Remember to breathe into the tight spaces in your body. Explore the interplay between your breath and the softening of the muscles around your shoulder blades.

There should be almost no effort on your part to rest in this position. If your knees struggles to reach the floor due to tight muscles, place a pillow underneath it for support.

If you experience pain anywhere in your body, gently come out of the pose, relax for around 30 seconds to a minute on your back, and then roll to one side and when you ready, stand up.

Laying Down Twist Pose Benefits

Physical Benefits

This exercise stretches your chest, obliques (abdominal), and glute muscles. The chest stretch is especially potent, as it promotes natural, deep breathing.

The twisting action of your spine helps to keep it flexible. It also creates more space between the vertebrae, allowing more hydration and improving spinal nerve function. This, in turn, improves the flow of energy throughout your body. As you do this pose, it stimulates the circulation of blood in your abdominal area, promoting the health of your digestive tract.

Emotional And Mental Benefits

This is a feel-good pose that relaxes your body and mind.

When To Avoid The Laying Down Twist Pose

- If you are pregnant.
- If you have had a spinal injury in the past, consult your doctor before attempting this pose.
- If you have a recent spinal injury, don't try this pose.
- If you have chronic digestive issues.
- Talk to your doctor first if you are prone to experiencing inflammation in your abdominal area.
- If you have a knee injury.
- If you have a hernia.
- If you have a slipped disk.

Self-Reflection

After doing the Laying Down Twist Pose, reflect on how you feel physically and emotionally.

Date:_____

_____
_____
_____
_____
_____
_____
_____
_____
_____
_____
_____
_____
_____
_____
_____
_____
_____

Corpse Pose (*Savasana*)

If your body had a reset button, this restorative Yoga pose would be it. With this regenerative pose, you'll learn to relax one body part at a time. Usually, when you first start practising this pose, one of two things will happen:

- You'll fall asleep.

- You'll stare at the ceiling, your thoughts racing all over the place, with a tense-feeling body.

Both are OK. Don't judge yourself. Instead, take your time to perfect the method because only time and persistence can teach you to be calm and at rest, even if you're awake. It's no easy thing to learn, so practise self-love—always.

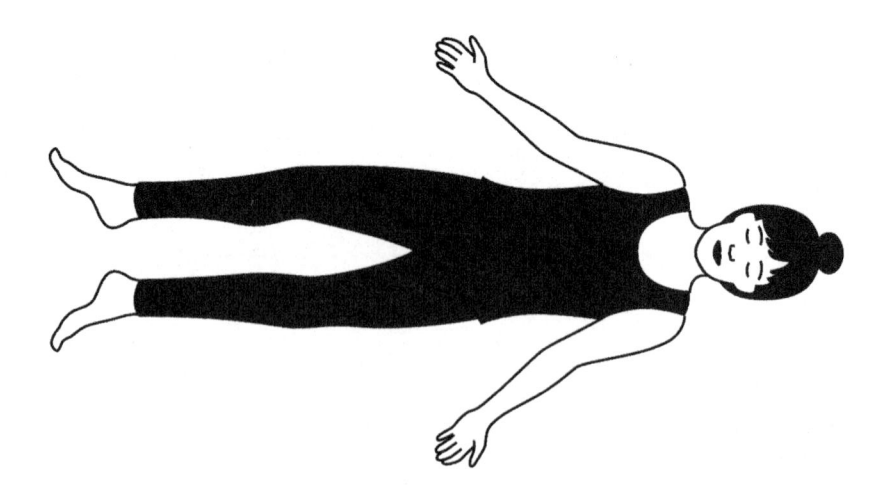

Self-Reflection

Before doing the Corpse Pose, reflect on how you feel physically and emotionally.

Date:_____

_____
_____
_____
_____
_____
_____
_____
_____
_____
_____
_____
_____
_____
_____
_____
_____
_____
_____

How To Do the Corpse Pose

Although you ideally want around 15 minutes for this technique, you'll probably stay in the pose for shorter lengths of time in the beginning—around 5 to 8 minutes. This is a good pose to do before bedtime, whenever you need a break, or when your love bundle wakes you and you can't fall asleep again.

You can do this pose with or without props. Common props include an eye bag or cloth over your eyes for added relaxation, a folded blanket resting horizontally over your abdominal area for added relaxation, a rolled-up towel or blanket under your knees to support your lower back, a folded towel or blanket under your head to support your neck, or a folded towel or blanket to support each of your wrists.

Note that this is normally the last pose you'll do at the end of a Yoga class. To get the most benefit out of being in this pose, try doing at least one of the other poses in this chapter first. You can also practice it after following an online Yoga class, for example.

Step 1

Lie down on your back. You might experience a bit of twitching, coldness, and discomfort the first few times. This is all part of the process of learning to relax, so allow your body to go through the motions.

Spread your legs out so they're about shoulder-width apart and let your arms rest comfortably next to your body, your palms face the ceiling.

Step 2

Draw your shoulders to the floor, toward your mid line, so your chest gently lifts and opens. Try not to move from position as you extend your body. Take a couple of deep breaths, pull it in as much as you can, and then release it completely. This signals to your nervous system that it's OK to relax.

Step 3

Draw all your attention inward, focusing on your heart rate and breath. As you breathe, mentally scan for and identify areas of tension in your body and release them. Start with your feet and work your way up. When you get to your pelvic area, relax it completely and imagine that your pelvic organs are relaxing with it. Concentrate especially on your lower and upper back muscles and release their tension. Relax your wrists, arms, shoulders- imagine them relaxing so much that they just melt into the floor. Next, focus on the facial muscles on your forehead, eyelids, temples, and cheeks. Let your tongue rest on the lower palate and release all the tension in your jaw, throat, and neck.

As this pose takes you deeper into a relaxation mode, imagine that all your muscles are so relaxed that it's impossible to lift them. Bring your attention to your breathing. You might notice that your breathing is very slow and quiet, which is an indicator that the practice is working for both your body and mind.

Step 4

To come out of the pose, start taking deeper breaths. Next, wiggle your fingers and toes, bring your knees up to your chest, and turn to rest on your right side. Take a minute or two to bring your mind back to a wakeful state while keeping your eyes closed. When you're ready, lift yourself into a sitting position with your legs crossed.

Variations of the Corpse Pose

Corpse Pose with Your Legs On a Chair

This variation is best to release abdominal tension and puts less strain on your lower back. With your calves resting on a sofa or chair, follow the same steps as with the regular corpse pose.

Corpse Pose Benefits

Physical Benefits

The corpse pose releases tension throughout your body, calms your nervous system, lowers blood pressure, and promotes a better quality of sleep.

Emotional and Benefits

With a relaxed body, your mind will naturally be more at ease. Since this pose also calms your nervous system, you'll become less reactive in stressful situations and feel better equipped to navigate daily frustrations constructively. As an added bonus, you can enjoy increased awareness and focus better on tasks that require a lot of mental effort.

When to Avoid the Corpse Pose

- If you have lower back issues, it's best to consult your doctor before attempting this pose.

- Don't practise the pose after the first trimester of your pregnancy.

- If you feel upset or recently experienced trauma, you may feel more comfortable doing this pose with your eyes open.

Self-Reflection

After doing the Corpse Pose, reflect on how you feel physically and emotionally.

Date:_____
_____
_____
_____
_____
_____
_____
_____
_____
_____
_____
_____
_____
_____
_____
_____
_____
_____
_____

Chapter 8
Yogic Sleep To The Rescue

When we got to know each other back in Chapter 1, I mentioned that life would never, ever be the same. The truth is, no mum will get back all those lost hours of sleep.

However, with the right mindset and tenacity, we can use tiny spaces of time to boost our energy reserves and take care of ourselves.

We are mums, after all, so tenacity flows through our veins!

From Grumpy To Chilled Mama In 30 Minutes

The last self-care method I want to share is called Yoga Nidra, or Yogic Sleep. On the days I feel too tired to be awake but too awake and occupied to take a nap, Yoga

Nidra is my energy-boosting, mood-improving trump card in my arsenal of self-care techniques.

The philosophy of Yoga Nidra is vast. To fully appreciate it and the way it can positively impact your daily life, you'd have to study the subject. While it is certainly deserving of being studied, I know that a mother only has so much time. Sometimes, all you want to hear is, 'This is how you can feel better', and that is what I want to give you.

So, instead of diving into the details of this wondrous practice, I'm going to give you an overview of what Yoga Nidra entails, its history, and how it can radically change your life from one characterised by exhaustion to one of a woman who looks and feels in control. After that, we'll dive into the important part: how to practise Yoga Nidra with a 15-minute guided practise.

What Is Yoga Nidra?

In essence, Yoga Nidra is a technique that allows your body to enter a restful state while your mind maintains a fine balance between a wakeful and sleepful state. A successful 20-30 min Yoga Nidra session is as effective as 2 hours of uninterrupted sleep.

Brain waves

During the sleeping cycle, which you learned about in Chapter 1, your brain waves change as you go through each stage. Note that your brain waves also change during the day, depending on your circumstances and how you feel. In fact, there is always harmony, a symphony of sorts, of waves working in your brain. For the sake of clarity, let's discuss brain waves in the context of the sleeping cycle since you are already familiar with it.

When you go to bed, you experience beta waves, which translates into a wakeful state during which your body and mind are both active and able to respond to external stimuli (like noise) in an instant. Next, you experience alpha waves. By the time this happens, your mind and body are in a relaxed state, and your brain also promotes the release of serotonin, an important hormone that regulates your mood.

As you enter the dreaming or REM stage of the sleeping cycle, your brain produces theta waves, relaxing your mind further but also enhancing its learning capacity. Your body is now in a restful state and will not easily respond to external stimuli. While your brain is in the state of producing theta waves, it also helps you get rid of stressful and negative thoughts or experiences. People who are experienced in meditation have the ability to tap into this state of consciousness at will. It is this ability that allows them to live a life characterised by less reactivity in frustrating situations and an increased capacity to shake off bad habits and form new, positive ones at a faster pace than people who do not practise meditation. Finally, during the deepest and most restorative stage of the sleeping cycle, your brain produces delta waves. When in this state, your brain suspends all external awareness, allowing your body and mind to get rid of toxins, heal itself, and rest so you can function at 100 per cent when you re-enter the wakeful state. Yoga Nidra taps into this state of consciousness, which is why I believe it is the ultimate restorative self-care ritual for new mums.

Yoga Nidra also helps you to tap into the realm of your unconscious and subconscious minds, the ultimate reckoning forces that influence your motivations and behaviours.

The unconscious mind stores your deepest motivations and behavioural patterns, which are mostly unknown to you. These deeply-held beliefs and drives, including some unprocessed experiences from different times in your life, all influence your subconscious mind. It, in turn, influences which thoughts and emotions enter your conscious mind and translate into behaviours. Your subconscious mind contains thoughts and memories you're not necessarily aware of at the moment. However, it is possible to access the subconscious mind to better understand yourself without being judgemental.

When practising Yoga Nidra, you enhance the receptivity of your mind, allowing your subconscious mind to come to the forefront while your conscious mind takes a step back. The ability to tap into your subconscious mind is powerful, as it gives you the opportunity to identify, address, and change some of the negative behavioural patterns stemming from your unconscious mind. I say 'some' because, technically, you will likely require in-person, therapeutic and professional guidance to fully access the motivations and behavioural patterns in your unconscious mind. Although you can definitely become more aware of, access, and change the things that enter your subconscious mind. In doing so, your subconscious mind will take the lead and help your conscious mind manifest new attitudes and behaviours. With practise, you can set yourself up to gain new knowledge faster, treat illnesses more effectively, boost your creativity and problem-solving skills, and become the most authentic version of yourself.

The History Of Yoga Nidra

Some say Yoga Nidra is as old as the Indian civilisation itself. It is indeed an ancient practice that can be traced back thousands of years, appearing in the earliest Hindu and Buddhist texts. The traditions that Yoga Nidra was a part of were considered very sacred and not meant for the public. Knowledge of these philosophies, traditions, and practices was passed on directly from teacher to student in the ancient world.

Yoga Nidra was an unknown practice until 1964 when Swami Satyananda Saraswati from the Bihar School of Yoga introduced it to the general public in an attempt to train his successor, Swami Niranjanananda Saraswati. However, the version he introduced was an adaptation of the original Yoga Nidra, his reason being that the newer generation of yogic practitioners' attention spans were decreasing because of how the world was changing. It might also be that he wanted to preserve the sacredness of the practice in its original form, but we'll probably never know.

Today, Yoga Nidra as we know it is an evolving discipline, but it remains a deeply relaxing and restorative self-care ritual at its core. In whichever way its techniques may change in the future, I believe the essence of what you can achieve with this practice will remain intact.

For the most part, Yoga Nidra is a guided exercise where a teacher will lead you through different stages using verbal instructions. While sessions generally last 30 to 45 minutes, I have developed 15-minute practises specifically for busy mums. We'll dive into one of them in the *Guided Yoga Nidra Practise* section.

How Yoga Nidra Helps You Sleep Better & Other Benefits

> ### Rest Bite Takeaway
>
> When done right, the rejuvenating effects of Yoga Nidra are truly astonishing. For that reason, please keep in mind that this technique is by no means a substitute for sleep; it is merely a tool to boost your energy levels and ability to live in the moment.
>
> With constant practise of this and the other self-care rituals you have learned, you will set yourself up for better quality sleep, no matter how little of it you get to enjoy.

In 2002, a study found that practising Yoga Nidra increased the practitioners' dopamine levels. This hormone, together with serotonin, plays an important role in regulating your sleep patterns. If there is an imbalance of dopamine and serotonin being produced in your body, restful sleep is very difficult (if not impossible) to achieve. A case study published in 2017 reported improved sleep and more daytime productivity for the participants who had been suffering from insomnia for many years. Then there are the many women, including those who come to my practice for guidance, who report that Yoga Nidra allows them to fall asleep and stay asleep with almost unbelievable ease. Another reason this method is so effective in helping you sleep is because when practising yogic sleep, you learn to release your thoughts. As you know, high stress levels and negative thoughts keep you up at night, so you need a way to steer your mind clear of them, especially at night. This is exactly what Yoga Nidra offers. The best part is that with regular practise, combined with the other self-care rituals in your arsenal, you can begin to take control of your thought patterns and enjoy more peace of mind every day, allowing you more mental space to enjoy every precious second with your child.

Other Health Benefits Of Yoga Nidra

- In some cases, Yoga Nidra has proven more effective in reducing stress and anxiety than regular meditation.

- Because you activate theta and delta waves during Yoga Nidra sessions, your body can heal and get rid of excess toxins. Regular practise can improve your memory and cognitive function, giving you more capacity to learn and focus.

- Practising Yoga Nidra has shown a boost in confidence and self-esteem in people who suffered physical injuries

- It can help to reduce chronic pain.

- If you struggle with menstrual fluctuations, you can help to regulate your cycles by practising Yoga Nidra.

- Improved immunity and physical health.

I have come to believe that caring for myself is not self-indulgent. Caring for myself is an act of survival.

(Andre Lorde)

Guided Yoga Nidra Practise

Although you can practise Yoga Nidra whenever you need it most, doing a session in the evening, shortly before bedtime, will put your body and mind in the restful state you need to get the most out of the time you sleep—even if your baby decides to wake you up in the middle of the night.

Before you start with the following guided practise, get yourself comfortable in the position best suited for practising Yoga Nidra by following these guidelines:

For this exercise to be effective, make sure you have a time slot minimum of 15 minutes in which you'll be undisturbed.

The goal is to be as comfortable as possible, as you'll stay in this position for at least 15 minutes. You can do this while sitting, but I recommend you lie down on the floor or on your bed (preferably on your back) and use props like a blanket for warmth or support under your knees.

Take deep breaths until you are focused on this moment only.

When you're ready, you can start the guided practise. While doing this, try to immerse yourself by focusing and following along every step of the way with the words that guide you. If you do this right, there is a fair chance you may emerge from your very first session feeling refreshed and rested. However, do not take on your first Yoga Nidra sessions with unrealistic expectations. As with most new things in life, it will take persistent practise to realise the full benefits this powerful self-care ritual offers.

Before you start your Yoga Nidra, close your eyes. Focus on your breathing.

Every time you inhale, allow that breath to flow down your entire body. Every time you exhale, be fully aware of how your body becomes stiller and more at ease. As your body settles into this stillness, allow your mind to follow.

Allow your body to transition into a deep resting state by keeping your mind focused on your breathing and the stillness your body feels. Let your mind slowly travel throughout your body, taking in every part as your breathing takes in and releases air.

Your body is still, resting deeply, but your mind is alert.

Take your attention to the right side of your body. Let it become aware of your right thumb, index finger, middle finger, ring finger, little finger... Move on to your right palm, the back of your hand, your wrist, your forearm, your elbow, your upper arm, your shoulder... Move down to your right side, waist, hip, buttock... Go to your upper right thigh, then the lower part. Move on to the top of your right knee, then the back. Go on to the top of your shin. Finally, move on to your right calf, ankle, heel, sole, the top of your foot, your big toe, second toe, third toe, fourth toe, and your little toe.

With your next inhalation, bring your awareness all the way to the top of your body and let your mind notice your head, right arm, left arm, right leg, and left leg.

Now let your mind's awareness go over your left thumb, index finger, middle finger, ring finger, little finger... Move on to your left palm, the back of your hand, your wrist, your forearm, your elbow, your upper arm, your shoulder... Move down your left side, waist, hip, buttock... Go to your upper left thigh, then the lower part. Move on to the top of your left knee, then the back. Go on to the top of your shin. Finally, move on to your left calf, ankle, heel, sole, the top of your foot, your big toe, second toe, third toe, fourth toe, and your little toe.

With your next inhalation, guide your awareness all the way to the top of your body and let your mind notice your head, right arm, left arm, right leg, left leg.

Let your awareness move on to the base of your spine, the small of your back, the middle parts of your back, the upper parts of your back... Become aware of your right shoulder blade, then your left shoulder blade...

Move on to the back of your neck, the back of your head, the top of your head, your forehead, your right temple, your left temple, your right eye, your left eye, your right ear, your left ear, your right cheek, your left cheek...

Now become aware of your nose, lips, tongue, chin...

Move on to your right collarbone, left collarbone, the right side of your chest, the left side of your chest, and the centre of your chest... Become aware of the upper part of your belly, your navel, the lower part of your belly, your right groin, your left groin, and your pubic bone.

Be fully aware of your whole body. Feel how it rests.

Draw your awareness to the feeling of heaviness. Feel your body becoming heavy, and notice this sensation all over, from your head to your fingers, all the way down the middle of your body, even your toes.

Now let that experience of heaviness go. Feel your body becoming so light it floats. Feel as light as a feather. Notice this sensation of weightlessness all over your body, from your head to your fingers, all the way down to the middle of your body, even your toes.

Let the experience of weightlessness go. Draw your attention to the feeling of coldness. Let your memories take you back to a time you experienced extreme coldness and let it fill you.

Release yourself from the experience of coldness and draw your attention to the feeling of warmth. Let the feeling of heat fill your entire body.

Let the experience of heat go. Bring all your awareness back to your breathing. Feel the air moving in and out of your nostrils and be fully aware of the smooth pace of the breath coming in and out of your body.

Push this awareness of breath to every part of your body, as if your entire body is breathing. Ease into the sensation of resting. Let every inhalation bring vitality to your body, and let every exhalation bring stillness and quietness. Be fully aware of the powerful capability of breath to nourish every inch of your body.

Take in the sound of your breathing. Let it fill you. Focus on the sound and let it become louder and louder until you can hear it entering and exiting your nostrils. Let the awareness of the sound of your breathing bring your body back to awareness with your mind, back to the beginning of this exercise.

Feel how your body has just woken up from a deep and intense healing rest. Your body and mind are now both refreshed and full of new energy.

Still aware of the sound of your breathing, let that awareness expand to your surroundings and allow your body to become wide awake. Wiggle your fingers and toes, stretch your hands, your feet, your arms, your legs, and extend your entire body in any way you feel comfortable.

After stretching, curl up and turn on your side. Take a moment and, when you're ready, sit up straight, eyes still closed. Become even more aware of the sounds and smells around you. When it feels just right, open your eyes.

Rest Bite Takeaway

As your child's mother, you are the sole source through which he receives nutrition for his body and nourishment for his mind. From the time your baby was in your womb, everything you listened to, ate, and experienced has impacted him/her. He will continue absorbing what he learns from you like a sponge, so this is the perfect time to introduce him/her to the importance of caring for himself/herself to live a balanced life through your own actions.

Conclusion

Ah, motherhood.

What a weird, scary, and wonderful thing.

I'll be honest: as a first-time mum, you have many challenges ahead with your little love bundle, but overwhelming exhaustion will not be one of them because you have the secret to beating it. Exhaustion should not steal your joy again.

You've come a long way since the first chapter, and I'd like to commend you for loving yourself enough to take action. Too many mums out there believe the wellness and happiness of their households, families, and even friends are more important than their own. They push their own pain, exhaustion, and fears far, far away when interacting with others. But when they're alone, where no one can see them, they have to look themselves in the mirror and face the inevitable: they're miserable, and they don't know how to escape that dreaded feeling that they're not in control.

If there's one thing I hope you have not only realised but accepted, it is that your well-being and happiness *are* important.

If you don't prioritise your well-being, you cannot possibly give your all to your partner and child. So, if you're still not convinced that you need to take care of yourself for yourself, then do it for them. If you want the best for your baby, then you have to be at your best: well rested, focused, and present in every precious moment.

Let's recap what you have learned from Rest Bites:

Health and Wellness Start and End with Quality Rest

You now understand the sleeping cycle and how being able to go through just one complete cycle at night can help you wake up refreshed. That's not to say that's all you need to escape the exhaustion, but it's a start. You also know that your baby's sleeping cycle differs from your own, and being aware of when she wakes up and sleeps will give you an opportunity to nap during the day to recharge your batteries.

Prioritise rest because your mind and body depend on it. I shared scientific evidence to show you that the only time your brain clears itself of toxins is when you sleep. If you neglect sleep, you risk developing health complications that can affect you physically and mentally.

There's No Going Back

As they say: out with the old, in with the new. This is your life now, and it is a hundredfold better than where you came from, despite the interrupted sleep and frustrating moments. These days will pass. And believe it or not, you'll look back at them with a nostalgic heart.

The best thing to do is accept that life will never be the same again and to adapt to a new, better way.

Unchecked Stress is Destructive

Stress is a part of life, and it definitely has its place. That does not mean you should allow it to overwhelm you, though. If you can't recognise and manage stress effectively, you risk falling prey to anxiety, depression, and other stress-related health issues. More than that, stress is contagious. Before you even realise it, it can spill over to your partner and even to your baby.

You also explored the concept of parenting stress. In my humble opinion, parenting stress is a given and not really possible to avoid. However, if you're aware of its presence in your life, as well as its effects on you and your child, you can implement strategies to minimise it. As you know now, research shows that there is brain wave and heart rhythm synchrony between you and your baby. Since you are the one through whom your baby learns to communicate and connect with other people, you should do everything you can to minimise parenting stress (and stress in general), as this will ensure that he has the best chance of healthy cognitive and emotional development.

Pay Attention to Your Body's Signals and Make Self-Care a Priority

When you experience physical pain or discomfort, your body is telling you that something is wrong. It's a cry for help, a warning that you need to take better care of yourself. You learned about the concept of self-care and why it is important, the crucial reason being that taking care of yourself helps you regain your focus so you can engage in meaningful interactions with your child.

Self-care includes being honest with yourself about your mental and emotional well-being and having the willingness to engage in open, truthful conversations with those closest to you to help them understand how you feel.

Too many mums (and people in general) treat self-care as a selfish indulgence and fail to see how, in reality, it should be a way of life for everyone because their sanity and health depend on it. Treating self-care as a way of life turns it into a priority, and this requires forming positive, lasting habits.

Practise Self-Care Rituals Daily

From Chapters 4 to 8, you learned about the power of mindfulness, meditation, touch, acupressure, Restorative Yoga, and Yogic Sleep (or Yoga Nidra). I showed you these concepts through the lens of science, my experiences as a first-time mum, and the experiences of the women I have helped. You also have access to several self-care rituals, designed especially for busy mums, within each of those chapters.

Remember that you need not practise all of them, nor is it necessary to rigorously stick to any one method if you don't connect with it. Experiment with the ones that 'talk' to you to find the best rituals for your personal circumstances. That said, know that persistence and consistency is the key that will deliver results in everything you do.

Share the Love

Thank you for spending time with me and for trusting me to show you the way to a better, happier life as a new mum. If you practise the habits and self-care rituals I introduced you to, you'll surely experience significant changes and finally kick the exhaustion out the door.

If you found this book helpful, please take a moment to share your honest opinion on your favourite book review platforms, such as Amazon or Goodreads. Your feedback could help another new mum find hope, too. After all, showing kindness and compassion to others is also a powerful way to reduce your stress levels and enhance your emotional well-being. That other mum may never meet you, but she may make a life-changing decision to prioritise her self-care—all thanks to you.

Finally, **here's to *you***, the woman who conquered her fears and chose to give her very best to her children every day.

About the Author

Just like you, Lucie Mala is a busy mum—the one who's

responsible for everyday stuff... The bills, the shopping, the nappies, laundry, jobs... But, amid all that, she has reclaimed herself and lives every day with thriving energy, joy, and calmness.

Before becoming a mum, Lucie had devoted her life to learning and teaching ancient restorative practices she had discovered 20 years ago. Out of sheer new-mum frustration, she decided to apply the knowledge of Yoga, Acupressure, and other ancient hands-on self-care practices she had gained from studying in the UK, India, and Thailand to motherhood.

Lucie is a pragmatist. She's a mum first, and everything else comes after that. But she also refuses to disappear under the duty and busyness of daily life.

Since her transition into motherhood, she developed even more passion to inspire other women to find the power of rest. She spreads the knowledge about reclaiming our nervous system to represent something powerful in our homes, communities, and in life.

Connect with Lucie on Instagram @the_rest_bites or on her website at TheRestBites.com.

Bibliography

Chapter 1 References

About sleep. (2020, December 8). Raising Children Network. https://raisingchildren.net.au/ newborns/sleep/understanding-sleep/about-sleep

Boyes, A. (2018, February 12). *6 Benefits of an Uncluttered Space—The psychology behind organizing and decluttering.* Psychology Today. https://www.psychologytoday.com/us/blog/in-prac tice/201802/6-benefits-uncluttered-space

Brain Basics: Understanding Sleep | National Institute of Neurological Disorders and Stroke. (2022, July 25). National Institute of Neurological Disorders and Stroke. https://www.ninds.nih.gov/health-information/patient-caregiver-education/brain-basics-understanding-sleep

Breus, M. (2022a, May 20). *What Time Should I Go to Bed? (And Why it Should be Before Midnight).* The Sleep Doctor. https://thesleepdoctor.com/sleep-faqs/what-time-shouldyou-go-to-bed/

Breus, M. (2022b, July 15). *How Long Should You Nap?* The Sleep Doctor. https://thesleepdoc tor.com/napping/how-long-is-the-ideal-nap/

Chaunie Brusie. (2020, August 25). *Which Essential Oils Promote Better Sleep?* Healthline. https://www.healthline.com/health/healthy-sleep/essential-oils-for-sleep

Cherney, K. (2019, November 14). *What's the Best Time to Sleep and Wake Up?* Healthline. https://www.healthline.com/health/best-time-to-sleep

Dewar, G. (2022, March 11). *Baby sleep patterns: An evidence-based guide.* PARENTING SCIENCE. https://parentingscience.com/baby-sleep-patterns/

Dhand, R., & Sohal, H. (2007). Good sleep, bad sleep! The role of daytime naps in healthy adults. *Current Opinion in Internal Medicine*, 6(1), 91–94. https://doi.org/10.1097/01.mcp.0000245703.92311.do

Durlach, J., Pages, N., Bac, P., Bara, M., & Guiet-Bara, A. (2002, March). *Biorhythms and possible central regulation of magnesium status, phototherapy, darkness therapy and chronopathological forms of magnesium depletion.* PubMed. https://pubmed.ncbi.nlm.nih.gov/12030424/

Hill, R. A. D. (2020, May 14). *Should You Drink Milk Before Bed?* Healthline. https://www. healthline.com/nutrition/drinking-milk-before-bed#effect-on-weight

Jacobson, B. H., Boolani, A., & Smith, D. B. (2009, March). *Changes in back pain, sleep quality, and perceived stress after introduction of new bedding systems.* PubMed. https://pubmed.ncbi. nlm.nih.gov/19646380/

Jacobson, K. (2020, May 1). *Stages of Sleep: NREM Sleep vs REM Sleep.* The Community to Sleep Care Professionals. https://www.aastweb.org/blog/stages-of-sleep-nrem-deepsleep-vs-rem-sleep

Lockley, S. W., Brainard, G. C., & Czeisler, C. A. (2003). High Sensitivity of the Human Circadian Melatonin Rhythm to

Resetting by Short Wavelength Light. *The Journal of Clinical Endocrinology & Metabolism, 88*(9), 4502–4505. https://doi.org/10.1210/jc.2003030570

Magazine, S. (2003, October 1). *The Stubborn Scientist Who Unraveled A Mystery of the Night.* Smithsonian Magazine. https://www.smithsonianmag.com/science-nature/the-stubborn-scientist-who-unraveled-a-mystery-of-the-night-91514538/

Magnesium in diet. (n.d.). Medline Plus. https://medlineplus.gov/ency/article/002423.htm

Magnesium-Rich Food Information. (n.d.). Cleveland Clinic. https://my.clevelandclinic.org/health/articles/15650-magnesium-rich-food

Mann, D. (2009, December 30). *Is Lack of Sleep Causing You to Gain Weight?* WebMD. https://www.webmd.com/sleep-disorders/features/lack-of-sleep-weight-gain

Okamoto-Mizuno, K., & Mizuno, K. (2012). Effects of thermal environment on sleep and circadian rhythm. *Journal of Physiological Anthropology, 31*(1). https://doi.org/10.1186/1880-6805-31-14

Pacheco, D. (2022a, April 20). *Does Warm Milk Help You Sleep?* Sleep Foundation. https://www.sleepfoundation.org/nutrition/does-warm-milk-help-you-sleep

Pacheco, D. (2022b, May 5). *Sleep Deprivation and Postpartum Depression.* Sleep Foundation.

https://www.sleepfoundation.org/pregnancy/sleep-deprivation-and-postpartumdepression

Pacheco, D. (2022c, June 10). *Postpartum Insomnia.* Sleep Foundation. https://www.sleepfoun dation.org/insomnia/postpartum-insomnia

Paturel, M.S., M.P.H., A. (2014, March). *The Benefits of Sleep for Brain Health.* Brain and Life.

https://www.brainandlife.org/articles/could-getting-more-high-quality-sleep-protectthe-brain/

Peuhkuri, K., Sihvola, N., & Korpela, R. (2012). Dietary factors and fluctuating levels of melatonin. *Food & Nutrition Research*, 56(1), 17252. https://doi.org/10.3402/fnr.v56i0. 17252

REM sleep vital for young brains | WSU Research | Washington State University. (2016, February 19). Washington State University. https://research.wsu.edu/2016/02/19/rem-sleep-vitalfor-young-brains/

Saxbe, D. E., Schetter, C. D., Guardino, C. M., Ramey, S. L., Shalowitz, M. U., Thorp, J., & Vance, M. (2016). Sleep Quality Predicts Persistence of Parental Postpartum Depressive Symptoms and Transmission of Depressive Symptoms from Mothers to Fathers. *Annals of Behavioral Medicine*, 50(6), 862–875. https://doi.org/10.1007/s12160-016-9815-7

The Science of Sleep: Understanding What Happens When You Sleep. (2021, August 8). Johns Hopkins Medicine. https://www.hopkinsmedicine.org/health/wellness-and-prevention/ the-science-of-sleep-understanding-what-happens-when-you-sleep

Suni, E. (2022a, April 20). *How to Design the Ideal Bedroom for Sleep.* Sleep Foundation. https:// www.sleepfoundation.org/

bedroom-environment/how-to-design-the-ideal-bedroom-forsleep

Suni, E. (2022b, April 22). *Nutrition and Sleep*. Sleep Foundation. https://www.sleepfounda tion.org/nutrition

Suni, E. (2022c, June 10). *The Relationship Between Sex and Sleep*. Sleep Foundation. https:// www.sleepfoundation.org/physical-health/sex-sleep

Suni, E. (2022d, August 10). *Stages of Sleep*. Sleep Foundation. https://www.sleepfoundation. org/stages-of-sleep

Taheri, M., & Arabameri, E. (2012). The Effect of Sleep Deprivation on Choice Reaction Time and Anaerobic Power of College Student Athletes. *Asian Journal of Sports Medicine*, 3(1). https://doi.org/10.5812/asjsm.34719

Wilson, N., Wynter, K., Fisher, J., & Bei, B. (2018). Related but different: distinguishing postpartum depression and fatigue among women seeking help for unsettled infant behaviours. *BMC Psychiatry*, 18(1). https://doi.org/10.1186/s12888-018-1892-7

Chapter 2 References

Dewar, G. (2022a, March 14). *Parenting stress: 12 evidence-based tips for making life better*. PARENTING SCIENCE. Retrieved September 14, 2022, from https://parenting science.com/parenting-stress-evidence-based-tips/

Dewar, G. (2022b, March 14). *Parenting stress: What causes it, and how does it change us?* PARENTING SCIENCE. Retrieved September 14, 2022, from https://parenting science.com/parenting-stress/

Dewar, G. (2022c, May 29). *Talking to babies: How friendly eye contact can make infants tune in — and mirror your brain waves.* PARENTING SCIENCE. Retrieved September 14, 2022, from https://parentingscience.com/talking-to-babies/

Fry, A. (2022a, June 24). *Stress and Insomnia.* Sleep Foundation. Retrieved September 14, 2022, from https://www.sleepfoundation.org/insomnia/stress-and-insomnia

Fry, A. (2022b, June 24). *Stress and Insomnia.* Sleep Foundation. Retrieved September 15, 2022, from https://www.sleepfoundation.org/insomnia/stress-and-insomnia

Headaches: Reduce stress to prevent the pain. (2022, August 9). Mayo Clinic. Retrieved September 15, 2022, from https://www.mayoclinic.org/diseases-conditions/tension-headache/indepth/headaches/art-20046707

Luca, S. I. (2021). *Brain Synchrony in Competition and Collaboration During Multiuser NeurofeedbackBased Gaming.* Frontiers. Retrieved September 14, 2022, from https://www.frontiersin.org/articles/10.3389/fnrgo.2021.749009/full

Mcleod, S. (n.d.). *Stress, Illness and the Immune System | Simply Psychology.* Retrieved September 15, 2022, from https://www.simplypsychology.org/stress-immune.html

Neuropeak Pro. (2022, April 22). *How Stress and Anxiety Affect the Brain.* Retrieved September 15, 2022, from https://www.neuropeakpro.com/how-stress-and-anxiety-affect-thebrain/

Robertson, R., PhD. (2020, August 20). *The Gut-Brain Connection: How it Works and The Role of Nutrition.* Healthline.

Retrieved September 14, 2022, from https://www.healthline.com/ nutrition/gut-brain-connection

Signs of Low Self-Esteem. (2020, November 25). WebMD. Retrieved September 15, 2022, from https://www.webmd.com/mental-health/signs-low-self-esteem

Stress Leads to Bad Decisions. Here's How to Avoid Them. (2018, January 31). Harvard Business Review. Retrieved September 15, 2022, from https://hbr.org/2017/08/stress-leads-tobad-decisions-heres-how-to-avoid-them

Stress Symptoms: Effects of Stress on the Body. (n.d.). WebMD. Retrieved September 14, 2022, from https://www.webmd.com/balance/stress-management/stress-symptoms-effect s_of-stress-on-the-body

Tension Headaches: Symptoms, Causes, & Treatments. (n.d.). Cleveland Clinic. Retrieved September 15, 2022, from https://my.clevelandclinic.org/health/diseases/8257tension-type-headaches

Valencia, A. L., & Froese, T. (2020, January 1). What binds us? Inter-brain neural synchronization and its implications for theories of human consciousness. *Neuroscience of Consciousness*, 2020(1). https://doi.org/10.1093/nc/niaa010

Why Eustress Is Good for You. (2022, May 11). Verywell Mind. Retrieved September 14, 2022, from https://www.verywellmind.com/what-you-need-to-know-about-eustress-3145109

Why Good Leaders Make Bad Decisions. (2019, February 7). Harvard Business Review. Retrieved September 15, 2022, from https://hbr.org/2009/02/why-good-leaders-make-bad-decisions

Chapter 3 References

Shinn. (2021, May 5). *Psychologically Speaking: Is My Baby's Emotional Intelligence On Track?* Variations. Retrieved September 15, 2022, from https://www.variationspsychology.com/ blogs/is-my-babys-emotional-intelligence-on-track

Chapter 4 References

8 Ways You Can Cope With Mommy Brain. (2020, March 26). Verywell Family. Retrieved September 15, 2022, from https://www.verywellfamily.com/what-is-mom-brain4774384

Ackerman, C. E., MA. (2022, September 10). *What Is Self-Awareness? (+5 Ways to Be More SelfAware)*. PositivePsychology.com. Retrieved September 15, 2022, from https://positivepsychology.com/self-awareness-matters-how-you-can-be-more-self-aware/

Bahrami F, Yousefi N. Females are more anxious than males: a metacognitive perspective. Iran J Psychiatry Behav Sci. 2011 Fall;5(2):83-90. PMID: 24644451; PMCID: PMC3939970.

Bertin, M. (2021, November 16). *A Daily Mindful Walking Practice.* Mindful. Retrieved September 15, 2022, from https://www.mindful.org/daily-mindful-walking-practice/ Bullock, G. B., PhD. (2022, January 18). *How Your Breath Controls Your Mood and Attention.* Mindful. Retrieved September 15, 2022, from https://www.mindful.org/how-yourbreath-controls-your-mood-and-attention/

Goyal, M., Singh, S., Sibinga, E. M. S., Gould, N. F., Rowland-Seymour, A., Sharma, R., Berger, Z., Sleicher, D., Maron, D. D., Shihab, H. M., Ranasinghe, P. D., Linn, S., Saha, S., Bass, E. B., & Haythornthwaite, J. A. (2014, March 1). Meditation Programs for Psychological Stress and Well-being. *JAMA Internal Medicine*, 174(3), 357. https://doi. org/10.1001/jamainternmed.2013.13018

Hwang, W. J., Lee, T. Y., Lim, K. O., Bae, D., Kwak, S., Park, H. Y., & Kwon, J. S. (2017, August 29). The effects of four days of intensive mindfulness meditation training (Templestay program) on resilience to stress: a randomized controlled trial. *Psychology, Health &Amp; Medicine*, 23(5), 497–504. https://doi.org/10.1080/13548506.2017.1363400 Mead, E. B. (2022, July 22). *The History and Origin of Meditation*. PositivePsychology.com. Retrieved September 15, 2022, from https://positivepsychology.com/history-ofmeditation/

Meditation: A simple, fast way to reduce stress. (2022, April 29). Mayo Clinic. Retrieved September 15, 2022, from https://www.mayoclinic.org/tests-procedures/meditation/in-depth/ meditation/art-20045858

Norris, C. J., Creem, D., Hendler, R., & Kober, H. (2018, August 6). Brief Mindfulness Meditation Improves Attention in Novices: Evidence From ERPs and Moderation by Neuroticism. *Frontiers in Human Neuroscience*, 12. https://doi.org/10.3389/fnhum.2018.00315

Pacheco, D. (2022, April 19). *How Meditation Can Treat Insomnia*. Sleep Foundation. Retrieved September 15, 2022, from https://www.sleepfoundation.org/insomnia/treatment/meditation

Riopel, L. M. (2022, September 13). *Mindfulness and the Brain: What Does Neuroscience Say?* PositivePsychology.com. Retrieved September 15, 2022, from https://positivepsychology.com/mindfulness-brain-research-neuroscience/

Team, M. (2021, December 22). *Physical & Mental Benefits of Meditation.* Mindworks Meditation. Retrieved September 15, 2022, from https://mindworks.org/blog/physicalmental-benefits-of-meditation/

The Benefits of Meditation for Stress Management. (2022, April 20). Verywell Mind. Retrieved September 15, 2022, from https://www.verywellmind.com/meditation-4157199

Thorpe, M., MD PhD. (2020a, October 27). *12 Science-Based Benefits of Meditation.* Healthline. Retrieved September 15, 2022, from https://www.healthline.com/nutrition/12-benefits-of-meditation#9.-Improves-sleep

Chapter 5 references

Cascio, C. J., Moore, D., & McGlone, F. (2019, February). Social touch and human development. *Developmental Cognitive Neuroscience, 35,* 5–11. https://doi.org/10.1016/j.dcn.2018.04.009

Cassata, C. (2018, June 27). *How Touching Your Partner Can Make Both of You Healthier.* Healthline. Retrieved September 15, 2022, from https://www.healthline.com/health-news/how-touching-your-partner-can-make-both-of-you-healthier

Goyal, M., Singh, S., Sibinga, E. M. S., Gould, N. F., Rowland-Seymour, A., Sharma, R., Berger, Z., Sleicher, D., Maron, D. D., Shihab, H. M., Ranasinghe, P. D., Linn, S., Saha, S., Bass, E. B., & Haythornthwaite, J. A. (2014, March 1). Meditation Programs for Psychological Stress and Well-being. *JAMA Internal*

Medicine, 174(3), 357. https://doi. org/10.1001/jamainternmed.2013.13018

Hwang, W. J., Lee, T. Y., Lim, K. O., Bae, D., Kwak, S., Park, H. Y., & Kwon, J. S. (2017, August 29). The effects of four days of intensive mindfulness meditation training (Templestay program) on resilience to stress: a randomized controlled trial. *Psychology, Health &Amp; Medicine, 23*(5), 497–504. https://doi.org/10.1080/13548506.2017.1363400

Mayer, B. A. (2021, September 28). *Does Your Body Have Energy Channels? Here's What the Science Says.* Healthline. Retrieved September 15, 2022, from https://www.healthline.com/health/mind-body/does-your-body-have-channels#channels-101

Morales-Brown, L. (2021, January 20). *What does it mean to be "touch starved"?* Retrieved September 15, 2022, from https://www.medicalnewstoday.com/articles/touch-starved

Norris, C. J., Creem, D., Hendler, R., & Kober, H. (2018, August 6). Brief Mindfulness Meditation Improves Attention in Novices: Evidence From ERPs and Moderation by Neuroticism. *Frontiers in Human Neuroscience, 12.* https://doi.org/10.3389/fnhum.2018. 00315

Chapter 6 References

Acupressure. The Gale Encyclopedia of Senior Health: A Guide for Seniors and Their Caregivers. . Retrieved August 25, 2022 from Encyclopedia.com: https://www.encyclo pedia.com/caregiving/encyclopedias-almanacs-transcripts-and-maps/acupressure

Johnson, J. (2018, May 17). *What is a qi deficiency?* Retrieved September 15, 2022, from https://www.medicalnewstoday.com/articles/321841

Lu, D. P., & Lu, G. P. (2013, October). An Historical Review and Perspective on the Impact of Acupuncture on U.S. Medicine and Society. *Medical Acupuncture*, 25(5), 311–316.

https://doi.org/10.1089/acu.2012.0921

Skuban, S. F. C. R. M. T. /. (n.d.). *What Are the Benefits of Acupressure? | Massage School Miami.* Retrieved September 15, 2022, from https://www.amcollege.edu/blog/benefits-acupressure-massage

Team, C. (2018, June 8). *Top 5 benefits of acupressure.* Colorado Pain Care. Retrieved September 15, 2022, from https://coloradopaincare.com/blog-top-5-benefitsacupressure/

White, A. (2004, January 27). A brief history of acupuncture. *Rheumatology*, 43(5), 662–663. https://doi.org/10.1093/rheumatology/keg005

Zhang, W. B., Wang, G. J., & Fuxe, K. (2015). Classic and Modern Meridian Studies: A Review of Low Hydraulic Resistance Channels along Meridians and Their Relevance for Therapeutic Effects in Traditional Chinese Medicine. *Evidence-Based Complementary and Alternative Medicine*, 2015, 1–14. https://doi.org/10.1155/2015/410979

Chapter 7 References

Ezrin, S. (2021, December 14). *16 Benefits of Yoga That Are Supported by Science.* Healthline. Retrieved September 16, 2022, from https://www.healthline.com/nutrition/13-bene fits-of-yoga

Nichols, H. (2021, April 15). *How does yoga work?* Retrieved September 16, 2022, from https://www.medicalnewstoday.com/articles/286745

Chapter 8 References

Adams, A. (2021, January 9). *8 Benefits of Yoga Nidra: Reduce Stress, Improve Sleep...* Ambuja Yoga. Retrieved September 16, 2022, from https://ambujayoga.com/blog/benefits-ofyoga-nidra/

Datta, K., Tripathi, M. & Mallick, H.N. *Yoga Nidra*: An innovative approach for management of chronic insomnia- A case report. *Sleep Science Practice* 1, 7 (2017). https://doi. org/10.1186/s41606-017-0009-4

Ferreira-Vorkapic, C., Borba-Pinheiro, C. J., Marchioro, M., & Santana, D. (2018). The Impact of *Yoga Nidra* and Seated Meditation on the Mental Health of College Professors. *International journal of yoga*, 11(3), 215–223. https://doi.org/10.4103/ijoy.IJOY_57_17

Kjaer, T. W., Bertelsen, C., Piccini, P., Brooks, D., Alving, J., & Lou, H. C. (2002, April). Increased dopamine tone during meditation-induced change of consciousness. *Cognitive Brain Research*, 13(2), 255–259. https://doi.org/10.1016/s0926-6410(01)00106-9

Luminescent, T. (2020, September 1). *YOGANIDRĀ*. Retrieved September 16, 2022, from https://www.theluminescent.org/2015/01/yoganidra.html

Posted by:YOGA.IN TEAM. (2019, November 12). *An Introduction to the Roots of Yoga Nidra*. Yoga in India. Retrieved September 16, 2022, from https://blog.yoga.in/2019/11/12/an-introduction-to-the-roots-of-yoga-nidra/

Yoga Nidra for Sleep: How Yogic Sleep Can Help Improve Sleep Hygiene. (2022, February 1). Retrieved

September 16, 2022, from https://www.anahana.com/en/yoga/yoga-nidra-for-sleep

Printed in Great Britain
by Amazon